FRIEDMAN'S FABLES

Friedman's fables

Edwin H. Friedman

THE GUILFORD PRESS
New York   London

© 1990 The Guilford Press
A Division of Guilford Publications, Inc.
72 Spring Street, New York, NY 10012

Printed in the United States of America

This book is printed on acid-free paper.

Last digit is print number: 9 8 7 6 5 4

Library of Congress Cataloging-in-Publication Data
Friedman, Edwin H.
   (Fables)
   Friedman's fables / by Edwin H. Friedman.
      p.   cm.
   ISBN 0-89862-440-1
   1. Conduct of life.   2. Interpersonal relations.   3. Interpersonal
communication.   I. Title.   II. Title: Fables.
BF637.C5F75   1990   90-47336
158'.2—dc20   CIP

Book design by Denise Adler

Illustrations by Joseph Cavalieri and Stephen Wilder

These fables are dedicated to the tutors of my imagination:

*The English Department of Bucknell University—
for cultivating my love for metaphor*

*Rabbinic Midrash—for teaching me how playfulness
can turn irreverence into an act of faith*

*Dr. Murray Bowen—for opening my eyes to the
protoplasmic unity of creation*

*My mother's wit—she was the quickest
one-liner I ever met*

Contents

God invented man because he loves stories.

Prologue

Introducing the Author
and His Characters

The publication of these fables took longer than expected. The delay began when the publisher gave them to a stylist. He jazzed them up, but the glitz clouded the primitive naiveté essential to this art form like the shadow thrown by a developing cataract. I was horrified. Next, various members of the staff tried to help, and they varied in their opinion about every single one. I became confused. Finally, they were given to a rewrite man, who wanted me to rewrite them. I offered to return my advance. Though I also began to realize that the fables were already doing exactly what they were supposed to do—engage readers personally and stimulate their own imaginative powers.

I was, however, a little surprised at the depth of

my own reactions. Why was I taking such umbrage? At first I thought it was the form. After all, how would you like it if your still-life was criticized on the basis of how the flowers were arranged? Next I thought it was the plots. What right, I thought, has anyone to criticize your story because of the story you chose? But later I saw it was the characters. Over the years, as I had read these fables to clients and to audiences, they had become my companions. They were not merely my creations but, ultimately, as I have tried to show in the Epilogue, my partners in creation. They had even influenced the development of one another. No wonder I was so angry; everyone was interfering with my relationships.

Then I remembered what Luigi Pirandello had written about his *Six Characters in Search of an Author*. After describing how they visited his mind one night and refused to go away until he gave their possessing presence stage for a separate existence, he wrote:

> Every creature of fantasy and art, in order to exist, must have his drama, that is, a drama in which he may be a character and for which he is a character. This is the character's *raison d'être*, his vital function, necessary for his existence. (*Naked Masks: Five Plays*, 1952, p. 368)

My experience with the characters in these fables was similar. Each entered my mind most unexpectedly and, once inside, surfaced repeatedly until I could finish their plot. Except, unlike Pirandello's experience, I had joined them as part of the cast. The usual result of long-term performances, of course, is that everyone develops a bond. In a very real sense, therefore, by publishing their stories I let my characters go and allow myself to experience the sadness and withdrawal that follows the break-up of any troupe.

There is a sweetness to the sadness, however, for my experience with my characters also differed from Pirandello's in a more fundamental way. Their initial visit never came in my solitude. It was always when I was in dialogue with some other. The context of their birth, every one of them, was when I was listening to another person's tale. Born of dialogue, the *raison d'être* of these characters is in their dialogic potential. Their "vital function" on this planet is to talk to the reader, and they fully expect to be talked back to. Not only that—as with the conditions of their birth, the reader will find that if introduced to others, privately or publicly, they are exceedingly adept at stimulating conversation. Indeed, perhaps because of the context of their being, they have a way of affecting bonds. This is the drama that is necessary for *their* existence.

An author's characters also act out his own drama, too, of course. The part of my story that is hidden here is the past three decades I have spent in the Washington metropolitan area, intimately involved in our species' three major systems of salvation: politics, religion, and psychotherapy. I have observed a whole generation go by of families, of governments, and of modes of therapy, all the while struggling to discern the illusion of change from the reality that things are pretty much the same as when I got here. The universality of this experience has left me wondering, Why has all the intelligence, and wisdom, and experience, and knowledge that has advanced our species in so many other areas of civilization not worked nearly as well in the improvement of our species itself? Is it that human nature is simply human nature? Are we

somehow all cursed? Or is it something more simple than
that, like the possibility that we are all caught up in myths
about what it takes to get others to hear? For everywhere
the paradox seems to be the same: Not only are com-
municants failing to listen to their mentors, they are ac-
tively tying their tongues.

The characters in these fables, therefore, also have
another role than the part they play in their own plot.
Their separate stories have been organized in such a way
that the network of their collective fantasies can drama-
tize the reality of that perversity. In this they are icono-
clasts, and the illusions they aim to shatter are:

- that communication is a cerebral phenomenon
  rather than an emotional process
- that insight will work with people who are unmotivated to change
- that resistance to your message can be overcome
  by trying harder
- that seriousness is deeper than playfulness

Sit back in your box, therefore, and let them strut their
stuff across the stage of your own imagination.

THE
FAILURE
OF
SYNTAX

The colossal misunderstanding of our time is the assumption that insight will work with people who are unmotivated to change. Communication does not depend on syntax, or eloquence, or rhetoric, or articulation but on the emotional context in which the message is being heard. People can only hear you when they are moving toward you, and they are not likely to when your words are pursuing them. Even the choicest words lose their power when they are used to overpower. Attitudes are the real figures of speech.

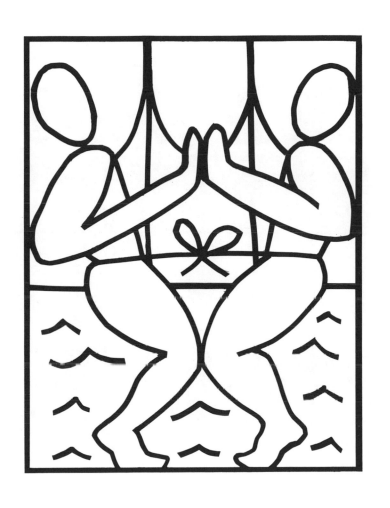

The Bridge

There was a man who had given much thought to what he wanted from life. He had experienced many moods and trials. He had experimented with different ways of living, and he had had his share of both success and failure. At last, he began to see clearly where he wanted to go.

Diligently, he searched for the right opportunity. Sometimes he came close, only to be pushed away. Often he applied all his strength and imagination, only to find the path hopelessly blocked. And then at last it came. But the opportunity would not wait. It would be made available only for a short time. If it were seen that he was not committed, the opportunity would not come again.

Eager to arrive, he started on his journey. With

each step, he wanted to move faster; with each thought about his goal, his heart beat quicker; with each vision of what lay ahead, he found renewed vigor. Strength that had left him since his early youth returned, and desires, all kinds of desires, reawakened from their long-dormant positions.

Hurrying along, he came upon a bridge that crossed through the middle of a town. It had been built high above a river in order to protect it from the floods of spring.

He started across. Then he noticed someone coming from the opposite direction. As they moved closer, it seemed as though the other were coming to greet him. He could see clearly, however, that he did not know this other, who was dressed similarly except for something tied around his waist.

When they were within hailing distance, he could see that what the other had about his waist was a rope. It was wrapped around him many times and probably, if extended, would reach a length of 30 feet.

The other began to uncurl the rope, and, just as they were coming close, the stranger said, "Pardon me, would you be so kind as to hold the end a moment?"

Surprised by this politely phrased but curious request, he agreed without a thought, reached out, and took it.

"Thank you," said the other, who then added, "two hands now, and remember, hold tight." Whereupon, the other jumped off the bridge.

Quickly, the free-falling body hurtled the distance of the rope's length, and from the bridge the man abruptly felt the pull. Instinctively, he held tight and was almost dragged over the side. He managed to brace himself against the edge, however, and after having caught his breath, looked down at the other dangling, close to oblivion.

"What are you trying to do?" he yelled.

"Just hold tight," said the other.

"This is ridiculous," the man thought and began trying to haul the other in. He could not get the leverage, however. It was as though the weight of the other person and the length of the rope had been carefully calculated in advance so that together they created a counterweight just beyond his strength to bring the other back to safety.

"Why did you do this?" the man called out.

"Remember," said the other, "if you let go, I will be lost."

"But I cannot pull you up," the man cried.

"I am your responsibility," said the other.

"Well, I did not ask for it," the man said.

"If you let go, I am lost," repeated the other.

He began to look around for help. But there was no one. How long would he have to wait? Why did this happen to befall him now, just as he was on the verge of true success? He examined the side, searching for a place to tie the rope. Some protrusion, perhaps, or maybe a hole in the boards. But the railing was unusually uniform in shape; there were no spaces between the boards. There was no way to get rid of this newfound burden, even temporarily.

"What do you want?" he asked the other hanging below.

"Just your help," the other answered.

"How can I help? I cannot pull you in, and there is no place to tie the rope so that I can go and find someone to help me help you."

"I know that. Just hang on; that will be enough. Tie the rope around your waist; it will be easier."

Fearing that his arms could not hold out much longer, he tied the rope around his waist.

"Why did you do this?" he asked again. "Don't you see what you have done? What possible purpose could you have had in mind?"

"Just remember," said the other, "my life is in your hands."

What should he do? "If I let go, all my life I will know that I let this other die. If I stay, I risk losing my momentum toward my own long-sought-after salvation. Either way this will haunt me forever." With ironic humor he thought to die himself, instantly, to jump off the bridge while still holding on. "That would teach this fool." But he wanted to live and to live life fully. "What a choice I have to make; how shall I ever decide?"

As time went by, still no one came. The critical moment of decision was drawing near. To show his commitment to his own goals, he would have to continue on his journey now. It was already almost too late to arrive in time. But what a terrible choice to have to make.

A new thought occurred to him. While he could not pull this other up solely by his own efforts, if the other would shorten the rope from his end by curling it around his waist again and again, together they could do it. Actually, the other could do it by himself, so long as he, standing on the bridge, kept it still and steady.

"Now listen," he shouted down. "I think I know how to save you." And he explained his plan.

But the other wasn't interested.

"You mean you won't help? But I told you I cannot pull you up myself, and I don't think I can hang on much longer either."

"You must try," the other shouted back in tears. "If you fail, I die."

The point of decision arrived. What should he do? "My life or this other's?" And then a new idea. A revelation. So new, in fact, it seemed heretical, so alien was it to his traditional way of thinking.

"I want you to listen carefully," he said, "because I mean what I am about to say. I will not accept the position of choice for your life, only for my own; the position of choice for your own life I hereby give back to you."

"What do you mean?" the other asked, afraid.

"I mean, simply, it's up to you. You decide which way this ends. I will become the counterweight. You do the pulling and bring yourself up. I will even tug a little from here." He began unwinding the rope from around his waist and braced himself anew against the side.

"You cannot mean what you say," the other shrieked. "You would not be so selfish. I am your responsibility. What could be so important that you would let someone die? Do not do this to me."

He waited a moment. There was no change in the tension of the rope.

"I accept your choice," he said, at last, and freed his hands.

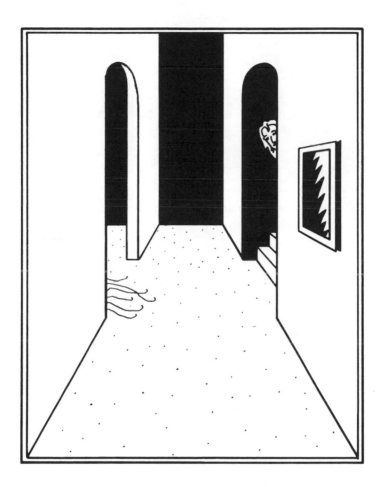

A Nervous Condition

When little John was about a year old, his parents noticed very thin fibers protruding through his pores. After another few months the fibers had extended themselves. They began to form curls. The condition alarmed his parents, so they took little John to a doctor. The physician, after examining him carefully, called in several specialists. They, in turn, summoned their colleagues and, after conferring for several hours, announced: Little John was unique in medical history—his ganglia were growing outside his skin.

Since there was no record of this having happened before, it was not clear what the ultimate effects of such a condition would be, and since little John was otherwise in excellent health, it was decided to do nothing for a while but observe.

Of course, one immediate problem was little John's rapidly developing, extreme sensitivity to everything and everyone around him. The doctors alerted his parents, warning them that they must be supersensitive to his every move and touch. Being very sensitive people anyway, they readily agreed.

As little John grew, so did his ganglia, until they trailed about him as he walked. While it was not a pretty sight, surprisingly it turned out to have some advantages.

He learned from the very beginning, for example, first from his ever-concerned parents and then from others, that he could always count on someone watching out for him. Indeed, he learned early in life that anyone who came into his orbit would always pay attention to his every move for fear of hurting him. He found that he could plough a path through any group of friends by just walking toward them. People would always retreat at his advance for fear of "stepping on his feelings." When he engaged in sports, or when he just wanted to be first in line, all he had to do was start in the direction he chose, and his approach itself proved to be an "open sesame."

Sometimes he encountered people who had not been forewarned about his condition, and then he had to point it out as early in their relationship as possible. Once they understood, however, they never tried to get in his way.

All of this is not to say that individuals never felt resentment toward little John. Some of his classmates, and one of his brothers in particular, who were most competitive with him for certain goals, felt handicapped by his handicap, but they never spoke it aloud. All managed to quiet their resentment with self-recriminations about their own insensitivity.

And so it went. Little John graduated high school (having done fewer homework assignments than any other child who ever attended), and he obtained a secure job, though less qualified than most of those seeking the same position.

One day he met a woman whom he liked. Being extremely shy and not having enough confidence or experience to refute her own poor image of herself, she was thrilled at the advances of this very attentive, if somewhat strange, creature. She treated him with the utmost deference, and her pity soon became love. Everywhere they went she watched out for him. In time, the guiding principle of her life became, "How can I help this man avoid pain?"

But after they had been married a while, she began to tire. Still she tried, for this poor man could not help himself. But it became increasingly difficult for her to be constantly mindful of his needs. She decided to confess her increasing insensitivity to her friends. She mentioned it to her family, to her minister, to her doctor. She sought professional help. All comforted her and sympathized but could offer little practical advice, and so they urged her to be more patient. She tried again to shape her existence to his needs. Then the headaches started. Then the little tic in her eye. Soon she found she was losing weight. Colitis further restricted her freedom, and it was not long before her thoughts were bordering on suicide. She dared not tell little John, of course, for fear of hurting him. Why, if he knew that all of this was due to his condition, he would be inconsolable.

One day, as she was walking home, she chanced

upon a mother cat giving suck to her newborn kittens. As they scrambled over one another in their thirst, the mother carefully guided each one to its turn, stretching out a firm but gentle paw as she lay contentedly on her side. Then little John's wife noticed that one of the kittens had been born lame; its leg had not been fully formed, and it had more difficulty maneuvering than the others. Strangely, it was also the most aggressive. While the other kittens, when satisfied, went off to sleep, this one kept coming back to wiggle its way in front of thirsty others. Each time, however, the mother cat pushed it away, at first gently, and then with successively harder whacks.

Little John's wife watched the poor kitty and the "inhuman" mother. But when she returned home, upon finding her husband reading in a room, she planted herself in the doorway and began to stare. A little while later, little John, desiring to enter another room, marched straight for the doorway that framed his wife. She did not budge. Closer he came, closer, never thinking actually to ask her to move (after all, he had never had to ask anyone to get out of his way before). Suddenly, he stopped, confused. What should he do? First he assumed his most wounded look. Then he tried one that was more winsome and boyish, but his wife was like a rock. In desperation, he finally spoke. "Move. You know I cannot squeeze by." Nothing. "What's the matter with you?" he yelled. "What are you trying to do to me? This is like a trap." Then she did begin to move, not aside, but rather directly toward him. He retreated. She continued on. He moved back faster, but still on she came. Soon he was cornered.

"Have you lost your mind?" he said incredulously. "Careful there, you almost hurt me," he said pathetically. That did it. She raised a foot and STOMP, with all her might she came down hard on one of his trailing nerve endings. He screeched, either from pain or shock. Again she stomped, and again and again. He ran past her, but she pursued. He screeched again, and the scream encouraged her more. STOMP, STOMP, she continued chasing him from room to room, up and down stairs, to the cellar, to the attic, through the kitchen, to their bedroom, until, exhausted, they both collapsed and fell asleep.

When Little John's wife awoke, her headache was gone for the first time in months. Her eye, too, had lost its quiver, and for the first time in a very long time she sighed without a pain and felt relaxed. But more astounding still was what she saw beside her. For, when she looked over at little John, she found that his ganglia were no longer curled around him all about the floor. On closer examination, she realized that they had disappeared altogether. In fact, they had completely recoiled inside his skin.

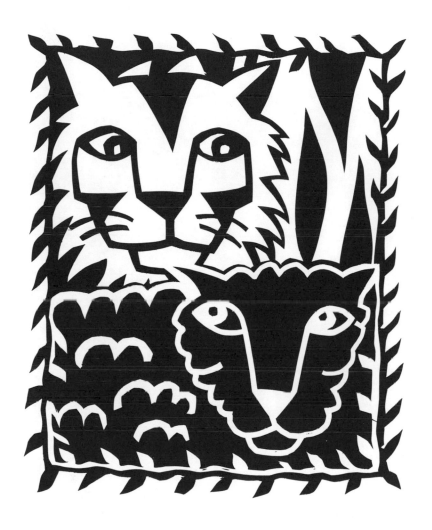

The Friendly Forest

Once upon a time in the Friendly Forest there lived a lamb who loved to graze and frolic about. One day a tiger came to the forest and said to the animals, "I would like to live among you." They were delighted. For, unlike some of the other forests, they had no tiger in their woods. The lamb, however, had some apprehensions, which, being a lamb, she sheepishly expressed to her friends. But, said they, "Do not worry, we will talk to the tiger and explain that one of the conditions for living in this forest is that you must also let the other animals live in the forest."

So the lamb went about her life as usual. But it was not long before the tiger began to growl and make threatening gestures and menacing motions. Each time the frightened lamb went to her friends and said, "It is very uncomfortable for me here in the forest." But her friends reassured her, "Do not worry; that's just the way tigers behave."

Every day, as she went about her life, the lamb tried to remember this advice, hoping that the tiger would find someone else to growl at. And it is probably correct to say that the tiger did not really spend all or even most of its time stalking the lamb. Still, the lamb found it increasingly difficult to remove the tiger from her thoughts. Sometimes she would just catch it out of the corner of her eye, but that seemed enough to disconcert her for the day, even if the cat were asleep. Soon the lamb found that she was actually looking for the tiger. Sometimes days or even weeks went by between its intrusive actions, yet, somehow, the tiger had succeeded in always being there. Eventually the tiger's existence became a part of the lamb's existence. When she tried to explain this to her friends, however, they pointed out that no harm had really befallen her and that perhaps she was just being too sensitive.

So the lamb again tried to put the tiger out of her mind. "Why," she said to herself, "should I let my relationship with just one member of the forest ruin my relationships with all the others?" But every now and then, usually when she was least prepared, the tiger would give her another start.

Finally the lamb could not take it anymore. She decided that, much as she loved the forest and her friends, more than she had ever loved any other forest or friends, the cost was too great. So she went to the other animals in the woods and said good-bye.

Her friends would not hear of it. "This is silly,"

they said. "Nothing has happened. You're still in one piece. You must remember that a tiger is a tiger," they repeated. "Surely this is the nicest forest in the world. We really like you very much. We would be very sad if you left." (Though it must be admitted that several of the animals were wondering what the lamb might be doing to contribute to the tiger's aggressiveness.)

Then, said two of the animals in the Friendly Forest, "Surely this whole thing can be worked out. We're all reasonable here. Stay calm. There is probably just some misunderstanding that can easily be resolved if we all sit down together and communicate." The lamb, however, had several misgivings about such a meeting. First of all, if her friends had explained away the tiger's behavior by saying it was simply a tiger's nature to behave that way, why did they now think that as a result of communication the tiger would be able to change that nature? Second, thought the lamb, such meetings, well intentioned as they might be, usually try to resolve problems through compromise. Now, while the tiger might agree to growl less, and indeed might succeed in reducing some of its aggressive behavior, what would she, the lamb, be expected to give up in return? Be more accepting of the tiger's growling? There was something wrong, thought the lamb, with the notion that an agreement is equal if the invasive creature agrees to be less invasive and the invaded one agrees to tolerate some invasiveness. She tried to explain this to her friends but, being reasonable animals, they assured her that the important thing was to keep communicating. Perhaps the tiger didn't understand the ways of a lamb. "Don't be so sheepish," they said. "Speak up strongly when it does these things."

Though one of the less subtle animals in the forest, more uncouth in expression and unconcerned about just who remained, was overheard to remark, "I never heard of anything so ridiculous. If you want a lamb and a tiger to live in the same forest, you don't try to make them communicate. You cage the bloody tiger."

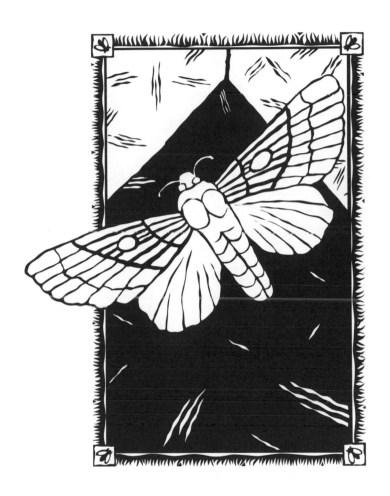

'Round in
Circles

Late one afternoon a moth emerged from its cocoon and chanced upon a fly buzzing about a window. With no particular purpose of its own, the moth was fascinated by the industry and vigorous intent of the other insect. Over and over, the fly would land on the pane, stay motionless for an indefinite time, and then suddenly, without any signal, retreat into the air, only to land inches away, after a short flight to nowhere in particular.

"What are you doing?" the moth asked.

"What do you mean, what am I doing?" answered the fly. "Can't you tell?"

"Well, I'm sorry," the moth replied. "It's just that

you seemed to be going about your business with such energy, and I was wondering . . ."

The fly landed a few centimeters away.

"I've been at this all day," he said, "and you want to know what I'm doing? Hmmmmf." And he took off again, flew for a few seconds, and returned, this time landing on the moth's other side.

"Look here," said the moth, rotating his whole body so he could see the fly better. "I just thought that maybe I could . . ."

But the fly had taken to the air again, as if never to return. He changed direction abruptly, however—in fact, it was so quick, it might have appeared to be one continuous flight—and descended further down the glass.

The moth glided over, landing gently nearby, but before he could continue his thought, the fly was once again in flight. Up he went, over and down, nearly a vertical descent this time, landing sharply to the left. Then, almost immediately, off, with a steep climb, but with a roundtrip that left him exactly where he had been.

"I really don't mean to be impolite," said the moth, "but I notice how you just keep taking off and landing. Yet you don't seem to be getting anywhere."

"Well, it won't help any talking to you," said the fly. "Time's a-wasting," he added, and elevated himself quickly, this time coming down at the top of the window.

Motionless, but ever intense, he called over to the moth. "Don't you realize that today is almost over?"— and then, without waiting for an answer, he flit. Though just as if he had been held to some limit by an elastic band, he rebounded upon the pane, circled to another spot, came back to the first, and finally stayed still, looking impassively on the softly swaying moth.

"Don't you ever get tired?" asked the moth.

"I can't allow myself to," said the fly as he bolted into the air, only to dart back to his previous position.

"What are you looking for?"

"Looking for?" the fly responded incredulously, then hurled himself out from the glass.

"You sure don't have much patience!"

"That's easy for you to say," the fly called back; then, hopping over, he added, "I only have today."

"The window's closed," said the moth.

"I know that!" replied the fly in a "don't be stupid" sort of way and zoomed off, circled, slowed almost to a hover, and quickly alighted nearby.

"I don't see any cracks or holes either."

"Tell me something new," the fly said sarcastically and took off.

When he had returned, the moth responded, "I mean there just doesn't seem to be any way at all to get to the other side."

"Look," said the fly, "I don't tell you how to run your life." And plummeting backwards from the window, he circled and touched down. "At least I try," he added after he had landed.

"God, you're serious."

"That's easy for you to say," the fly replied again, positioning himself for another take-off. "It's not your problem."

"But have you had any success?"

"Not yet; why do you think I have to keep trying?"

"How long will you continue?"

"Till I succeed."

"What if you don't?"

"I can't allow myself to think about that either."

"Suppose you cover every inch and still don't succeed?"

"I've already done that."

"You have? Then why don't you go to another window?"

"I can't do that. I have to keep trying."

"But you just said you've covered every inch."

"I might have missed something."

"At least," said the moth, "you might try another approach."

"I've considered that. I have decided to try harder." And as soon as he had announced his commitment, the fly rocketed away and began taking off and landing so frequently that he appeared to be bouncing off the surface.

"All those eyes sure don't help you to see much better, do they?" asked the moth.

"What do you mean by that?" returned the fly. He had come to a stop on the lower portion of the window.

"Well, I've been watching you, and maybe it's not how much one can see, but the angle."

"I've thought of that; why do you think I keep coming from a different direction?"

"I don't think you understand," said the moth. "I meant the attitude."

"I try as hard as I can."

"I meant perspective," said the moth with some exasperation. "You know, distance."

"I go a thousand times my height as it is. If I were

to go out any further, there would be less time left for landings."

The fly flew off again.

"Distance has to do with thinking!" shouted the moth, still trying to make the other understand.

"What's that?" asked the fly, intent on the glass window before him.

But the moth never heard the question. By now it had become dusk, and from somewhere far off, a light source began to radiate. The spark attracted its attention. Then, suddenly, as if by some secret command, the moth fluttered and took wing in the direction of the glow, where it crackled itself to a crisp on an electric arc.

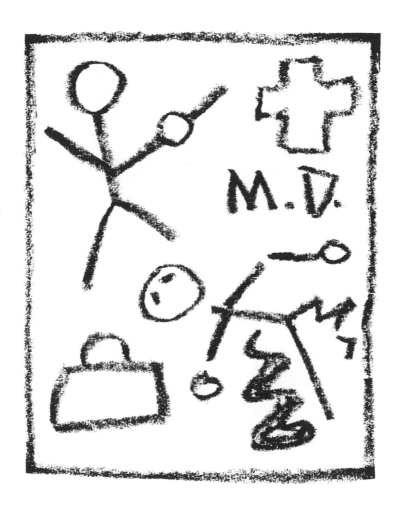

Projection

When Billy was about 6, he drew his first picture on the bedroom wall. His mother, torn between wanting her child to express himself and wanting her wall to be clean, decided to let him be.

As his hand grew more steady, however, Billy's mother noted that most of his drawings had something in common—all his figures were lying down.

Startled, she told her husband. After dinner, he went up to Billy's room. It was exactly as his wife had said. On each wall Billy had scribbled scenes of figures lying down. None of the figures were standing or sitting; everyone was lying down.

What could it mean? Should they ask him? Perhaps it was only a phase. Father thought it best to wait, but for Mother it became too difficult to avoid the subject completely. Finally, she said to her son, "Billy, I noticed that in all your pictures you always draw everyone lying down."

"Yes, mother," said Billy, and he went on drawing.

His mother was so upset by the sureness of her son's response, as well as his indifference to her anxiety, that, with the burning question now spoken, she dropped the subject and left the room.

After a month or so, however, as Billy's artistry improved, his mother noticed something else consistent in her son's drawings. Not only was everyone lying down, but it also appeared that everyone was hurt. Some seemed to have sticks protruding from their bodies; if faces were drawn, the eyes were always closed, and the position of many seemed to indicate that they were "out" or dead.

Again she told her husband, and again he found his wife was right. Each figure his son had drawn showed little life, and the ribbons of red color attached to many of the bodies suggested they were gushing blood.

Once more, the parents caucused. Why was their son fixated on pain? Was he trying to express his own? Was he depressed, maybe even suicidal? Perhaps he was angry. Late into the evening, his father and mother discussed possibilities. Were they not good to him? Had they unwittingly favored his sister? Had they failed to give him a chance to express his feelings? Should they consult a professional? "Oh, this is ridiculous," said his father, finally. "Why don't we just ask him?"

"But perhaps," worried his mother, "that's the worst thing we could do. I mean, to call attention to it. Suppose he is hiding things; he might bury them deeper."

Indecisive, Billy's parents went to bed to spend a sleepless night.

The next morning, however, Father walked into his son's room and said, with all the naturalness he could muster, "Billy, it seems to me that in each of your drawings, people not only are always lying down, but they also always seem to be in pain. I mean, is that how you meant it?"

"Yes, father," answered Billy, and said no more.

"Well," said his father, again trying hard to be natural, "just *why*, that is, how come . . . I mean, well, what's the reason for that?"

"That's just the way I think them up," said Billy, who continued playing with his toys.

As it had been with his wife, Billy's father became so disarmed by the nonchalance of his son's response that he dropped the subject and went to work. After all, Billy was basically a good boy. He never had trouble in school. Taking him to a doctor might actually nip something creative in the bud.

For the next half year, as Billy's artwork become more sophisticated, it could be seen that many figures actually had been in violent situations: run over by cars, hit on the head by rocks, stabbed, shot. His parents held their breath.

However, just around the time Billy turned 7, a new development occurred. Upon entering his room one afternoon, his mother noticed that the people in Billy's drawings no longer were whole. Limbs were missing, guts were hanging out, faces were smashed in, heads were severed. This was too much. Something sinister was clearly at work inside her son's head.

When her husband came home, she informed him

of her horrible discovery. What they found together was even worse. Not only were the people Billy drew torn to pieces, but so were his toys. Soldiers were missing arms and legs, a doll had its eyes ripped out, a stuffed cat was cut open at the belly.

That did it. His parents stumbled over one another to reach the phone. They obtained the name of a specialist in children's problems and hastily made the earliest appointment they could.

With the utmost caution, his parents explained to Billy that there was a nice man who wanted to talk to him, and 2 days later, after dressing Billy in his best clothes, they brought him over to the nice man for his interview.

He took their son into a separate room and asked him if he liked to draw. "Oh, yes," said Billy. Whereupon he produced some drawing paper and crayons and told the boy that he would be back in a little while. During that time, he assured Billy, that he was free to play with any of the toys in the room.

The specialist then left Billy and joined his parents in an adjoining room equipped with a one-way mirror.

Immediately, Billy set about drawing his people—lying down, scenes of violence, severed bodies. After a while he tired of drawing and began to play with some toy soldiers and dolls especially made to be pulled apart and rejoined. Immediately Billy began to break off the various parts and lay the mutilated remains side by side.

"See," said his parents, aghast, "it's just as we told you." Most alarming to the clinician, however, was the matter-of-fact attitude of the boy, the total absence of any feeling as he went about dismembering and then lining up the bodies.

The clinician told the parents to wait, entered the room where Billy was playing, and skillfully engaged him in harmless conversation around his play. Billy, as usual, always answered politely and to the point.

But the specialist found he could not get below the surface. He took a new tack. "Do you know what you want to be when you grow up?"

For the first time Billy showed some glee. "Oh, yes," said Billy.

Sensing success, he pursued the path. "I'm glad to see you can get excited. You know, your parents are afraid that you are a very angry child."

"Angry?" said Billy. "Why should I be angry? They are so nice to me. The only thing that would make me angry," continued Billy, "is if they would not let me be what I want to be when I grow up."

"And what is that?" the man asked, anxiously.

"A doctor!" shouted Billy, as he examined another severed toy.

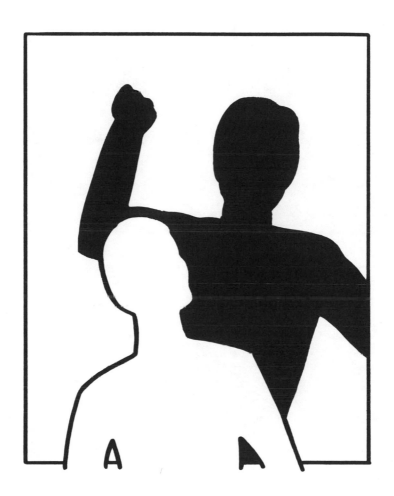

Raising Cain

A Case History of the First Family

Recent archeological discoveries have revealed a "family workup" done by one of the ministering angels about 20 years after Creation. It is translated here from the original.

This is a family of four: mother, father, and two sons, fairly close in age. They came in because the sons have been quarreling a great deal, and both mother and father appear quite helpless to do anything about it. Most of the focus is on the older brother, who broods a lot, is extremely sullen, and is very jealous of his far more successful younger brother.

The younger brother is not aware of his advantage and thus never tries to hide his success, his easy-going manner, or the rewards of his prosperity. The older seems totally unable to understand why fortune does not smile alike on him.

It cannot be said that the parents, both of whom are only children, by the way, show any significant favoritism. Yet I am quite sure it is something in their own style of life that is contributing to the very problem they want to solve.

At the beginning of their marriage, both husband and wife seemed to have lived in a very blissful state, naive, it appears, about what was happening all around them. Something, we're not sure what, changed that, and things have never been the same since. The husband growls continuously about his lot and why life has to be so difficult, whereas the wife never fails to remind him of how much pain she went through to bear him sons.

But it is more than their discontent that seems to be seeping down, particularly to their elder son. More pernicious still may be their attitude *toward* their discontent.

Neither husband nor wife seems capable of accepting responsibility for their own destiny. Both are always claiming that their lives would be far different were it not for how the other behaved. The man tends to blame his wife, and the wife tends to blame the environment.

But it is not only their own destinies that each sees as ruled by the other; they even view their own being similarly. Neither seems capable of taking responsibility for personal desires, loves, or hates. Each sees the other as causing his or her own pain. Ironically, they thus each give their partner great power to guilt the other.

Since neither talks much about their origins (they both seem to be cut off from their past), it is difficult to know how their own childhoods contributed to such irresponsibility, though there is a strong suspicion here that while they were growing up they had everything handed to them on a silver platter. Indeed, each seems to have led a youth totally absent of significant challenge.

This inability to deal with pain seems to have shown up almost as soon as they began to face any change at all. For example, the wife remembers quite vividly an instance in which her husband tried some new directions—tasting something new in life, I believe she called it—and, when this failed, held her responsible for showing him the opportunity. Of course she, for her part, instead of simply saying, "He still made the choice," also becomes defensive and blames the whole thing on some tricky character who, she claims, gave her the idea to begin with.

There seems to be no strength in the family at all, by which I mean the capacity of some member to say, *I am me, this is where I stand. I end here and you begin there,* etc.

It may be this constant expectation that the *other* should be *his* keeper that prevents each from taking responsibility for himself. And as long as this attitude persists in the parents, we can hardly expect the boys to act more pleasantly toward each another, still less at times to be watchful over the other. This situation will certainly leave a "mark" on one of them.

In a family like this, with no one able to tolerate his own solitariness, or, for that matter, anyone else's, I fear the weaknesses in the children will never be corrected. Actually, my fantasies are worse. For, if the current inability each parent manifests to deal with his or her own pain continues, I fear that Cain's view of life will never truly focus on himself and, perceiving the source of all his problems in his brother, he may one day up and kill him.

THE DEMONS OF RESISTANCE

The essential difficulty in trying to communicate with another is how to get past the interference of the resistance demons who inhabit that other. What makes this task especially difficult is that it is the intrinsic nature of such demons to stiffen in the face of efforts to will them away. Yet they often vanish on the spot when our own demons no longer resist them. When, rather than trying to assault those demons head-on, we can, instead, stimulate in others their own imaginative capacity, we can often subvert the contrariness of their demons from within. That is why all successful artists, no matter what their medium, are always careful not to give too much information to, or solve the problem for, the viewer.

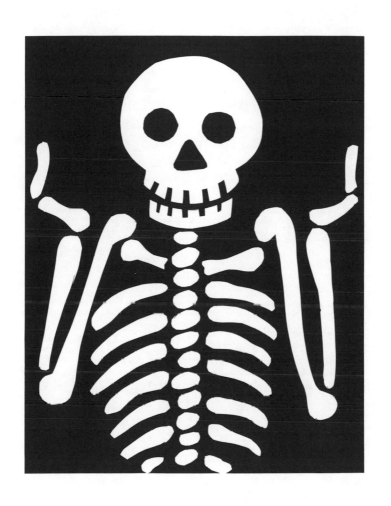

The Power
of Belief

One evening a man came
home and announced that he was dead.

Immediately, some of his neighbors tried to show
him how foolish this notion was. He walked, and dead
men cannot move themselves. He was thinking, his brain
was functioning, and he was breathing; and that, after
all, is the quintessence of living. But none of these argu-
ments had any effect.

No matter what reason was brought to bear against
his position, no matter how sensible the argument, the
man maintained that he was dead. He parried their thrusts
with ingenious skill.

He seemed to have a way of constantly putting
the burden of proof on the other. He never quite came

right out and said, "Prove it." But that was the message implied, not so much by how he answered as by how he avoided giving any answer at all.

Every now and then someone thought, "Now, I've pinned him down," having brought evidence so obvious no one could deny it. But then he would use his trump: "If I am dead, you do not exist either, since surely the living do not traffic with the dead."

Eventually most of his friends and neighbors quit arguing and the handful who were left, including his own family, became increasingly afraid.

Several reached the same conclusion: He had gone mad or, at the very least, was suffering from some erratic mental process. Exhaustion from work, perhaps? A brain tumor? He needs a rest, we'll call a doctor, perhaps a psychiatrist, maybe the family physician, or minister.

The man, however, was not upset by these suggestions. He shrugged them off without reply and finally said, "I don't know what's the matter with you all. It is just absurd to think of a dead man as tired, let alone sick."

His wife, almost literally beside herself, took to carrying on a dialogue within. ("If he believes this, then how can he say that? If he does that, how can he think this?")

As the mixture of fear and frustration thickened, it was finally agreed that outside help must be called. A psychiatrist was invited over to interview him.

After some preliminary greetings and a few routine questions, the doctor asked to see the man alone. He readily agreed. The two went into another room and closed the door. Now and then an elevated voice broadcast itself over the transom, although nothing could be understood. It was clear, however, that the voice they heard getting louder always belonged to the clinician.

Some time later, both men emerged. The doctor had his jacket over his arm, his necktie had been loosened and his collar opened (in fact, the button was no longer there). As for the man, he seemed totally unchanged. "Hopelessly psychotic," muttered the psychiatrist. "You will have to have him committed. He has lost all awareness of reality. If you want, I'll call the hospital and see if they have room."

"Now, really," said the man calmly, "what kind of therapy would you prescribe for a dead man? Surely, sir, if it were known that you had tried to cure a man who was not even alive . . . talk about losing one's grip on reality."

The doctor started to answer, caught himself, and then, with measured calm, said to the others, "I haven't finished dinner yet. If you want me to call the hospital, give me a ring."

A clergyman was sought. The family minister was unavalable. Which type would be best? The modern kind who had some sophistication about psychological problems? Or perhaps a good old-fashioned fundamentalist? "Let's fight fire with fire," said someone. As it happened, that evening a well-known evangelist was in town to speak at a nearby theater. When he heard about the problem he rushed over, thinking how his success might be used to introduce the show. Once again, the group was left to strain after the voices behind a closed door. Again, nothing that was audible, again the rising tone, again never the man's voice rising. This time the clergyman came out alone, stopped, looked at everyone, nervously kissed his little black book, and bolted out the door. Several cautiously peeked into the room; the man was fast asleep.

It was now decided that the family doctor should be called. He had known the man since he was a little boy, and besides being a physician with a reputation for patience and skill, he was respected everywhere for his homey wisdom. He came quickly, and after one or two questions in front of everyone, asked the man in a no-nonsense way, "Tell me, do dead men bleed?"

"Of course not," said the man.

"Then," said the doctor, "would you allow me to make a small cut in your arm, say above the elbow? I will treat it; there's no reason to worry about infection. I'll stop the flow immediately, and we can see, once and all, whether you are dead."

"Dead men do not get infections, nor do they bleed, doctor," said the man, as he proceeded to roll up his sleeve.

With everyone watching anxiously, the doctor deftly slit the flesh, and blood came spurting out. There was a gasp of joy throughout the group. Some laughed, others even applauded, though a few seemed rather to be relieved.

The doctor quickly dressed the wound and turned to everyone, saying, "Well, I hope that puts an end to this foolishness." Everyone was congratulating the physician when they suddenly realized that the man was headed for the door. As he opened it, he turned to the group and said, "I see that I was wrong." Then, as he turned to leave, he added, "Dead men, in fact, do bleed."

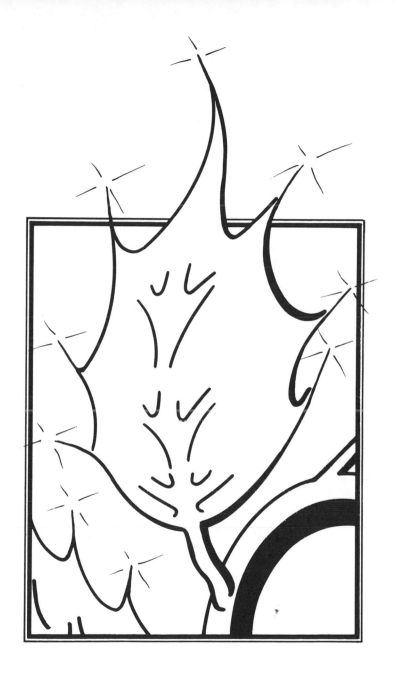

An American Holly

T here was a certain holly tree whose owner, when it was very young, planted it close to the foundation of his house to shelter the tree from the icy blasts of winter. He had done right. For it is the way of young, broad-leafed evergreens to lose their vital moisture to the evaporation of winter winds.

As time went by, however, the holly grew and soon found itself competing with that which had protected it during early life. The owner, therefore, decided to let the plant have more room. Carefully, early one spring, he dug up the sprouting tree and replanted it some distance away, so that it could branch out in all directions. As with the initial planting, the owner did everything with care; the roots were embalmed in a big ball of earth, a moat of mud surrounded the new site to keep the rainwater from running away, a deep protective blanket of the finest mulch covered the area about the slowly thickening trunk, and fertilizer, again only the finest grade, was liberally applied.

But all did not go well, despite the best intentions and the kindest care. The holly began to lose its leaves. Some were lost every year, of course, but others had always quickly blossomed to take their place. This time the dying leaves were not replenished. Something different was at work.

Perplexed by this unexpected turn of events, the owner gave his tree more care. He borrowed some books from the library to see what he could learn. He wrote to garden experts in the newspapers. Perhaps some blight or other noxious influence had come into the area, though he had read no warnings. He frequented the best garden shops and asked the old-timers what they did on such occasions.

Every question brought an answer; every question acquired more than one answer, if asked more than one time. And with each new suggestion, tale, or remedy he heard, the owner hurried back and tried anew. But nothing worked.

Each morning when the owner awoke he found that more leaves had fallen to the ground. Each week another branch was dead. Should these be allowed to remain on the trunk? Can life flow again through such hardened wood? Or does the dead decay and add decay to the living nearby?

When fall came, the holly was a sorry sight. Few leaves were left, and most of them were turning brown.

The frost came, and then it was too late in the year to try more remedies. But the owner hadn't ceased to care.

Every morning as he went to work, he saw the tree and wondered where he might have erred. Sometimes in the middle of the night, if he could not sleep and happened by the window, he would stop and stare. If there was moonlight, the branches, now so sparse of leaves, seemed even more bare.

Several times that winter it snowed, and the fall covered the lower, thicker part of the trunk so that the remainder looked like some cast-off limb that had fallen from a taller tree and javelined its way into the ground.

With the spring thaw, the holly's owner hoped again and waited for the buds. Perhaps with so few other leaves to share the nutrients, there would be more than ever. But no. If anything, there were fewer.

Still the owner tried: more fertilizer, a newer, softer blanket of mulch, further, careful pruning of the tips of the limbs, water with every day of sun. But the holly did not respond.

One day during the early summer, before the owner was about to leave for a vacation, he was preparing his other plants for some weeks without attention, and he came upon his sorrowful tree. Gingerly he pruned each little limb that had died. He would bend each back gently to see if the sign of life—the rubbery flexibility— was there, and, if so, he let it snap softly back into place; if not, with his clippers, as always, at the proper angle, he sheared it near the base, as always at the proper place. This time, however, something changed in his heart. Rather than pity, he began to feel anger.

Suddenly, he began to cut without checking carefully to be sure the limb was dead. Faster he began to clip, faster and with gusto, indiscriminately, this way and that, this limb and that, and then, in rage, the trunk itself. And, when he finally stopped, exhausted, his heart thumping, all that faced him was a scraggly stick that came up to his nose.

He hung his shears away and left with his family. Only once while they were gone did he think about the tree, and he said to his wife, "I'll dig it up when we return."

But when they returned something had changed. As they drove up, at first from the distance, and then with closer view, all could see the holly now bristling green. From every cut and wound and point from which a parted limb had gone, a hundred prickly, scorning tongues.

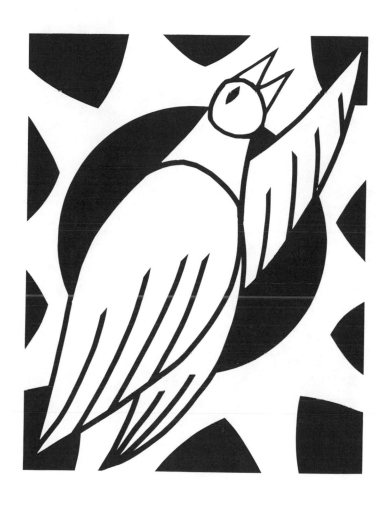

Soaring

Mr. and Mrs. Bird had successfully launched nine fledglings. Each had been hatched with no problems and grown to preflight performance with few complications. At the moment of "push-out," each had eagerly walked out on the ledge of the treehole in which their nest had been sheltered and, as their parents helped them clear the rim, spontaneously fluttered its wings in the most natural way. None seemed to need any special tutoring or coaching. All jumped out without any stalling whatsoever, fell a little, flapped a little, dipped, and flew.

Now, Mr. and Mrs. Bird were ready to leave the nest themselves. It had been their home a long time. Both were eager to spend their remaining years alone, to-

gether, satisfied that they had contributed to the survival
and the evolution of their species. As they had done nine
times before, therefore, they led Baby-Bird to the en-
trance of their shelter, and without too much thought
about it or concern, they gently pushed him out. Baby-
Bird at first fell a few feet just like his siblings before
him and then just kept on falling. In fact, he went into
an immediate nose dive, tail to the sky.

The Birds were alarmed. Mr. Bird could not believe what he was seeing.

"Flap your wings," cried Mrs. Bird.

"Pick your head up," shouted Mr. Bird.

"Fly! Fly!" they both echoed.

But Baby-Bird, nose to the ground, did not move
a muscle, nor did he seem to show fear. He did not call
back but just kept repeating to himself, "I'll be damned
if I'm going to flap my wings just 'cause they want me
to."

Further and further his little body plummeted
straight down like some plumb-line following a lead
weight.

"Loosen your feathers," cried his mother.

"Watch out," screamed his father.

Frantically they looked at each another; then, as
though they both had the same idea at once, each swooped
down on their offspring from opposite sides and caught
him before he was halfway down. They gently landed,
regained their strength, and flew him back to the nest,
chirping soothing noises all the way. "There, there, don't
be scared," or "Next time it will be easier," or "You just
have to get some confidence," or "We'll try again; tomor-
row will be better." But Baby-Bird did not respond; he
just kept thinking to himself, even more determinedly

than before, "I'll be damned if I'm going to flap my wings just 'cause they want me to."

The next morning Mama and Papa Bird tried again, this time a bit more anxious as a result of the previous day's experience. They went out of their way to comfort Baby-Bird, pointed out that it would be all right once he learned, and tried to raise his confidence by explaining how easily his brothers and sisters had done it before him. Mrs. Bird explained how to glide if he became tired, and Mr. Bird showed him how to flex his muscles more trimly.

Then, carefully, they set him on the rim of the hole again and, after a moment's hesitation, pushed. Baby-Bird went into a tumble.

"Fly," cried Mrs. Bird with far more anxiety than before.

"Move your wings," her mate followed, "your wings, your wings!"

But nothing his parents said had any effect on his "attitude" whatsoever. He just kept plummeting and thinking, "I'll be damned if I'm going to flap my wings just 'cause they want me to."

So, once again, Mr. and Mrs. Bird zoomed down from their perch, gently nestled themselves beneath his fall, decelerated slowly to the ground, and, after a brief rest, carried him back to the nest once more. The next day it was the same, and the day after that the same again. Days became weeks, and weeks became months. Soon the cold weather was approaching and likewise the winter of their lives.

Mama and Papa Bird were totally perplexed. What was wrong? They had never had any trouble with their previous children. What made matters worse was Baby-

Bird's refusal to help himself. He would not explain, refused to show any gratitude, and, if anything, became
more belligerent in proportion to their concern. The situation was even beginning to affect their own relationship. More than ever before they found that, if chirping
at Baby-Bird did not help, the resulting frustration found
them chirping at each another.

Then, one morning, Baby-Bird awoke. He heard
nothing. Usually he could hear his parents somewhere,
even if it was only the ruffling of their feathers. In fact,
that is generally what woke him up.

Normally, if he slept long enough, he could count
on one of them rushing in angrily, or, the opposite, coax-
ing him out with a rewarding morsel. But this morning
there was a peaceful, silent isolation. He tried to outwait
them as usual, but nothing happened. Finally he got
himself off his straw and went out of his cubicle.

He chirped. There was no response.

"They have gone out together? Most unusual."

He walked to the edge of the opening to see if he
could find them outside. It was a particularly beautiful
day, and the sky was seductively calling him. He re-
pressed the urge quickly, however, and ducked back in.
They were nowhere to be seen. He decided to go back
to bed and wait. But he could not sleep. He found himself anxious, fidgety. In the past he had always found his
parents' chirping a bother; he almost longed for it now.
Somehow those chirps and pokes had enabled him to avoid
his destiny, instead of facing it. He was beginning to
realize that much as he was annoyed by their calls, they
managed, in some way he could not comprehend, to take
the discomfort out of his indolence.

He became angry. "How dare they? Don't they

understand that I can't make it alone? Don't they care?" Finally, "I'll show them."

He went to the opening again. The ground was far away. Mama and Papa Bird had always made sure to put their nest high in a tree where it would be so much more secure.

He peered out over the edge of the hole in the bark. A trickle of fear ran through his otherwise cold-blooded body, but he quickly stopped it as he always did, with rage. "All the better. They'll never know what happened, and, if they do find out, maybe even come to see what's left, then they'll know, really know."

He resisted an urge to look around and dove out. He began tumbling as before, end over end, and he felt some loss of control. Then he stopped tumbling and angled straight for the earth below. He had hopes for a rapid descent and began to brace himself, eagerly, for the triumphal splat! When he was a little more than halfway down, however, further down than he had ever fallen before, something else uncontrollable happened. Both of his wings, simultaneously, and through no fault of his, pulled away from his body. He tried to tuck them back in, but air resistance prevented it. Worse, they proceeded slowly to span out further on both sides until they were fully extended.

The immediate effect, of course, was to pull Baby-Bird out of his nosedive. More, however, occurred than that. As his body gradually inclined upwards, his whole being felt an urge he had never sensed before. Caught in the flow of a gentle air current, he rose rapidly higher toward the clouds, and, for perhaps only the second time in his life, he looked at the sky.

The current carried him gracefully in a soft, elongated, parabolic curve, which, after it had borne him to its zenith, began to descend; and, inadvertently, again as if through no fault of his, he unwittingly, perhaps one could say instinctively, raised and lowered his wings.

Instantly his body stopped its short descent and he glided upwards again. He lowered and raised his wings once more, and once more his young, properly formed body moved effortlessly up in a graceful, inverted arc. The feeling was new, indescribably new. Riding the crest of his own energy now, he moved his head. Generally he was prone to look at his toes. He looked to the right, then to the left, and, as he tilted his head, found that even this movement affected his whole being, as he swooped up and over a flock of another feather.

His parents totally forgotten for the moment, and without their constant chirping to "foul" his functioning, he found, to his surprise, that he was able, almost naturally, to maintain the minimum velocity needed to prevent stalls. He experimented more.

Within no time at all Little-Bird was miles away. Looking around below, he could no longer locate his former home; there were trees everywhere. For a moment he wondered which had been his.

Then, with sudden resolve, he flapped his wings again and again, spurting and gliding upward. Out he went in new directions, diving, looping, turning, banking. One more time he remembered his nest, but with no vestige of his previous attitude. Oblivious, he soared to the sun.

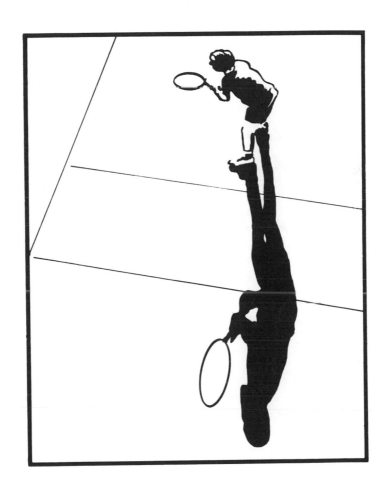

Net Results

One day, Harry decided to improve his wife's tennis game, not that she cared that much. First he found opportunities for her to learn; she never did. Next, he sent her to all the pros, but she did not progress. He bought her the latest how-to books, tapes of the champs; her game did not develop. He left magazine articles around in hopes she would read them. Her game remained consistent; though, curiously, she seemed to make better contact with her backhand.

As time went by, Harry's wife started to regress. She had more and more trouble getting up for it. Often, she would become sick just before a trip; sometimes she developed undefinable pains before a game. She fatigued easily. She began to withdraw. Then she hurt her arm,

after failing to follow through. It took her a year to recover.

When her arm got better, Harry decided to make
a breakthrough. He would teach his wife himself. First,
he bought her a new racket, taking special care to find
one that was well balanced, light, and with a grip she
would not find painful (as she had often complained). He
found shoes advertised not to make her feet sweat (something else that had bothered her), tennis shorts that were
not too long and not too short, and socks that were not
supposed to let her feet itch. He even bought balls with
extra bounce, frowned upon by many, including himself,
but if it would give her shots more oomph . . . And he
managed to find a court, mysteriously missed by others,
where they could play in seclusion and at a time that was
most convenient. His wife had often said that she did not
like others watching and that the hours when they could
usually reserve a court were not her best time of day. In
the end, Harry had nullified in advance every reason his
wife had ever given for why she had been distracted,
seemed listless, or was out of shape.

So one delightful morning, warm but not hot, with
only the slightest cooling breeze, he took his wife to the
out-of-the-way court. She did not seem overly excited
about the idea, in fact she developed a slight headache,
but she went. (On the way over, Harry realized she had
taken her old racket and had forgotten to wear the new
apparel he had bought her.) As soon as they got out on
the court, he walked his partner over to her position and
reviewed with her how to stand, how to place her feet,
how to bend her knees, how to hold her arms, her wrist,
her elbow, all the pointers he had gone over with her the
night before. Each time she silently allowed him to cor-

rect her stance, though once she did ask how long he thought they would be there.

He went over with her again how to hold the racket, how to anticipate a return, how to coordinate her timing, and then, enthusiastically, he ran back to his side of the court.

"Ready, dear?" he asked. And as soon as she nodded slightly, he softly hit a serve.

It passed her unmolested.

"What happened?"

"I wasn't ready."

He lobbed another. She barely moved but managed awkwardly to reach out and hit it back. The ball bounded into the net.

"What's the matter?"

"Just not up to it today," she said half-heartedly.

"I'm trying to help you, not hurt you."

"OK, OK," she said, "go ahead."

He was about to serve a third time when he noticed where she was standing. So he went back to her side of the net and positioned her once more.

"Set?" he asked, and without waiting for a response (which was not going to come anyway) he hit another, slightly harder than he intended. The ball bounced perfectly, however, almost homing in on her strings, and she returned the service. It zoomed off to her right, caromed off an old wooden bench, and ricocheted around in the corner between the rusty, green, grated fences until it became caught in the diamonds of the mesh.

Not wanting to discourage his wife, he shouted, "Good power, try to follow through a little more across your body."

"Don't you think we should paint the house this year rather than next?" she asked.

THWOCK! Harry's next serve headed for outer space. His wife had caught it at the very middle of her tether and sent it screaming over his head, over the iron mesh fence and beyond a large red maple on the other side.

"You really can put a lot on it," he yelled. "Try again."

SMASH! It came right back, a real zinger this time, smack into the middle of the net, where it bounced a few times and died.

"Good zip," Harry yelled, "try angling it up a little; I think you've almost got it."

Thus the volley continued. Harry would remind his wife how to stand, run over to her side of the court to demonstrate some principles of racket technique, run back to his side of the court to prepare for some dreamed-of reciprocity, initiate the dialogue with a clean, well-placed serve. And his wife would randomly send the ball its own willful way.

"Don't you want to play?" he asked finally.

She gave a slight shrug with her shoulders.

"You don't seem interested."

"Well, this was your idea, you know."

"Yes, but it's for you, that is, us . . . ," Harry broke off.

He knew, of course, that the game was more than skill or physical prowess. He was fully aware that playing well involved many emotional factors as well—self-control, for example, self-esteem, self-reliance. That playing well included the capacity to be assertive yet regulate one's intensity. That at the bottom of success was the mental toughness to respond well to challenge, the capacity to deal with adversity, to recover under pressure and somehow to maintain a positive attitude, to be bold, to take risks, and to be optimistic. These attributes were not only necessary for playing well; they were also the lessons the game could teach. He decided, therefore, to be the kind of teacher who was sympathetic, neither too overinvolved nor too critical, who was encouraging, and who remained supportive no matter what. He resolved never to guilt her and always to show he still loved her despite her faults. For he wanted her to feel valued, and, after all, the ultimate end was not how she ranked but fun.

He decided on a new tack. "She needs more guidance during the act itself," he thought. Harry served a high lob, underhanded, designed to bounce up right before her. Then he ran around to her side of the court, turned her shoulders in the right direction, held her arm with his hand, and guided the racket with just the right angle and speed to lob it back. He took off again, beat the ball to his side of the court, and lobbed it once again to hers, ran back behind her, held her arm just right, and guided the racket in a true path once more. Again, he started back to his side of the net, but it wasn't necessary. The ball had hit the racket wood and bounced aimlessly away.

He tried his new approach once more. Lobbed the ball, beat it to the other side, held her arm just right, and aimed the racket true. It crashed the net again. The next time, trying to correct for the previous fault, they sent it completely over the baseline, and a third time she wasn't ready, so that even together they missed making any contact at all.

He stood at his end of the court, dumbfounded,

reminding himself of his vows of patience. His wife stood at her end, wondering when she'd be out of the sun. What would it take to improve her game? He had taught her all the theory, all about technique; he had insured the best surroundings, obtained the finest equipment; she possessed all the natural resources.

Then, suddenly, Harry stopped asking. Slowly, he began to walk in a little circle. He bounced the ball vigorously a few times, wiped his racket handle of any sweat, positioned himself properly for a serve, and then, after glancing slightly to his right and to his left, he hit it with all his might, not directly toward his wife but up. Up and up it rose, and when it came down on her side, he was over there himself, ready for the return. Up he hit it toward his own side; he was back when it came down. Once more he batted the ball high into the blue so that he might have time to get under the return. So their match continued, forever and a day. And never again did Harry let it bounce on her end of the court.

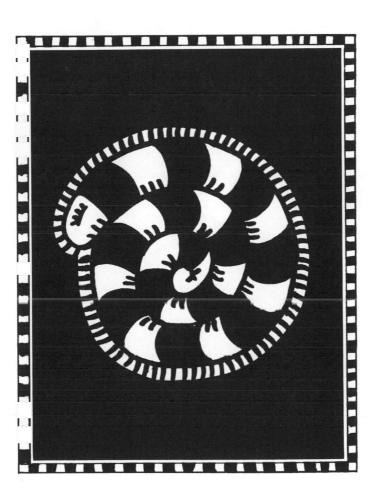

Metamorphosis

One morning Mrs. K. awoke and found that her husband had been transformed into a caterpillar. He was moving about slowly in the corner of the room usually reserved for the floor lamp, which had been sent out to be fixed.

Understanding immediately that this would necessitate changes in their marriage, Mrs. K. walked softly over to where the insect was standing and, trying carefully not to frighten him, reached over and began to caress his fur.

As soon as Mrs. K. touched him, however, the caterpillar curled up and refused to move. Surprised by the response, Mrs. K. tried to stroke her husband more gently and then, very slowly, tried to uncurl him. But he stiffened.

"There, there," she said. "I'm not going to hurt you. Don't be afraid." The caterpillar was unmoved.

Mrs. K. tried again. "I still care," she said. "We can still be close," she continued, whereupon she cupped the palm of her hand so as to provide a snug, cradle-like saucer. This would enable her husband to feel safe yet at the same time also allow him to straighten out. She let her hand roll a little to see if she could jar him into moving, but the caterpillar's response was totally passive. He simply let himself slide with the motion of her hand. At one point the caterpillar almost slipped over the edge of her fingers—he was still curled in a fur-like ball—so that Mrs. K. had to bring her other hand up quickly to make sure her husband didn't fall.

After this fright, however, her mood began to change. "Please," Mrs. K. implored. "Try to understand our situation. This is not going to be easy at all. I'm trying my best. The least I could expect from you is some acceptance." Still she felt no response. In fact, he seemed even more rigid than before.

She placed him down on the floor and continued to talk. "Perhaps," she thought, "if I did not hold on so tight he would show some sign of life." But the caterpillar remained still. "Would you like something to eat?" she asked, never asking herself what she would bring him. "You know, I'm going to have to go out pretty soon, and I'm somewhat afraid to leave you here all alone." Her husband remained impassive.

"Perhaps it's too cold in here," she thought, and, taking her husband in her hand again, Mrs. K. walked over to the window left ajar for the morning air and closed it tight. "There, you see, now it will be more pleasant."

She returned to the corner where she had first found him and tore a large leaf from a plant near the couch, placed it neatly on the floor, and gingerly put her husband down on the leaf to see if a more natural habitat would stimulate a response. But still the caterpillar did not budge. Her mood changed again.

"You know," said Mrs. K. a little testily, "I think I've been willing to adapt more than most women, but you can't expect me to go on like this if you are not going to be more cooperative." Nothing. "I'm not even asking you to speak. Good God, I don't even know if you can anymore! And I'm not saying you have to. But I need to have some idea of what you want. I mean, you can't leave this all up to me. Would you prefer to be in a box?" And so Mrs. K. continued talking to her husband until she began to wonder if she was only talking to herself.

Again she picked up her husband. He seemed to be even stiffer. Suddenly she put him right in front of her, at eye level, and squeezed. Nothing. Resisting, somehow, the urge to squeeze harder, she reached down and with a small stick began to poke the caterpillar. First she just touched him lightly to see if he would stir. Nothing. She prodded him harder. The caterpillar allowed himself to be rolled over by the poke. Then Mrs. K. began systematically to probe. Perhaps there was a soft spot, an area that was more vulnerable, and she began to examine her husband's furrows lengthwise along his body, taking care not to touch the head. Then she probed perpendicularly along the dark contoured circles. Neither the position of the poke nor the degree of force elicited a response. The caterpillar reeled or rolled back according to how Mrs. K. pushed. Not a single movement of the caterpillar could with certainty have been ascribed to his own will. Finally, fearful that she might hurt him, Mrs. K. dropped the stick.

Her husband was now curled so tight that no light could be seen coming through the coil. The thought ran through Mrs. K. that she had killed him. How would she know? There was no blood. Would he get cold if he was dead? She picked up the stick again and poked him one more time. Still, nothing.

Mrs. K. tried to assess her situation. It was clear that she must now take responsibility for everything, though that would not be too different from before. She would, of course, do all the work around the house, and unless it turned out that her husband could, in fact, talk, she would continue to take all initiative in their relationship. Camaraderie, not that there had been that much in the past, was clearly out of the question. On the other hand, if he would at least be willing to move a little on his own, that would certainly help.

Mrs. K. went into her closet, where she found a large shoebox. She took the top and folded back its edges so that it could serve as a ramp, went outside and gathered grass and leaves, placed a few aphids under a stick, and brought everything back to the corner of her bedroom that was to become her husband's place. She set the box down, put the ramp into position, and tried to show her husband how he could use the cover to get into the box. "Look, honey," she said soothingly. "I've made you a place where you can be secure. I'll try to change the leaves every day, and, while I don't know yet what you eat, I'll try to find out. The library must have a book on caterpillars." She picked her husband up again and, anticipating that he would begin to crawl along her arm, placed him on her lap. Nothing. The caterpillar just lay there on its side, curled in an oval, asleep or maybe dead.

Over the next several weeks Mrs. K. learned to adapt to the change. She continued to care for her husband, although he showed no response. The only way she knew he wasn't dead was that whenever she left the room for long periods of time, the caterpillar, upon her return, would always be in a different part of his box. However, in her presence he never moved.

Noticing this fact, Mrs. K. often pretended to go away, but, once having left the room, she would peer back from behind the door, hiding herself carefully so that the caterpillar could not sense her presence. Sometimes she would stay this way for hours. But he never showed any signs of life. Yet, at other times, she could be away for only minutes, and by the time she returned, the caterpillar had made his way completely to the other side of its box.

Eventually, whether through boredom or fatigue, Mrs. K. found herself thinking less and less about her husband. This bothered her in some ways, yet the freedom it engendered enabled her to return to thinking about herself. Then she received an invitation from an old friend to visit for a while. At first she said no. How could she leave her husband alone for so long? But at her friend's urging, she finally accepted, and after taking great care to put the box in a protected place, high on a closet shelf, filled with grass for comfort and for food, she left her husband alone for the first time in years.

During that visit, she completely stopped thinking about him. In fact, when she finally returned home, it was several days before she remembered the box. Quickly she rushed to the closet and anxiously looked in. The caterpillar was gone.

Had he been eaten? Could he have gone away? She was remonstrating with herself about her failure to be more concerned when the front door suddenly opened. There he stood, her husband, in the flesh. Mrs. K. could not believe her eyes. He rushed over to her, kissed her passionately, embracing Mrs. K. with a firm affection she had not experienced since their earliest days together.

"My God," he said, "where have you been? I thought I'd lost you."

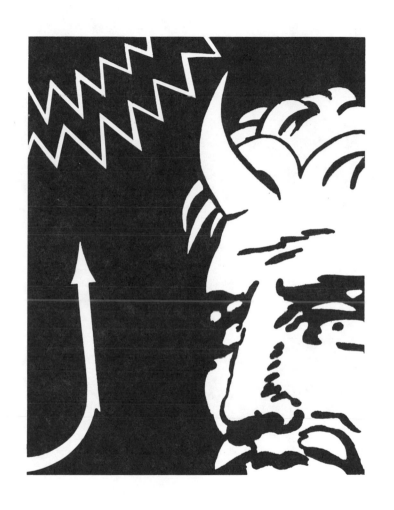

The Curse

Shortly after man and woman had been expelled from the garden of innocence, the Holy One turned to his favorite messenger and said, "Satan, I need a curse."

"What kind?" asked his servant.

"One that will last forever," replied the Master of Creation.

"That will be difficult," Satan responded.

"I know," said the Holy One. "That's why I've come to you. This one will require all your ingenuity and skill. It must get to the very essence of human existence, transcending culture and era."

"What went wrong with the first one?" asked the Prince of Darkness.

"There was nothing wrong with the idea," said the Lord of All, "but it turns out that some of these creatures actually love to work by the sweat of their brow."

"I'll get right on it."

Six days later, Satan returned. "My committee has been discussing this without pause. Every time we thought we had found it, we realized there was a flaw in the plan. It's very hard to encumber these new creatures in any permanent way," he continued. "Very persistent, you know; that life force is really something. But finally we found the perfect solution. Our problem was that we kept trying to fight the life force instead of going with it. Here's the idea: As we know, what most differentiates these creatures from the lower forms is that they have far more capacity for deep emotional bonds, due in part to their higher intellects, the length of the early dependence periods, etc. Anyway, it just hit us, why not create a way for those bonds to turn into binds?"

"Terrific," said the Lord of All. "How is it to be done?"

Satan grinned, then added tersely, "No one will marry the person that is good for them." He went on to explain. "Everyone will marry the one who brings out the worst in them; weaknesses and vulnerabilities will be the real lures. Everyone will choose a mate based on their bad habits rather than their good ones. No one will choose a partner who challenges them to grow. Everyone will choose mates who play into the very games they're used to playing, instead of being attracted to those who strengthen their own assets. But here's the best part. It will all be done unwittingly in a fog that resembles love but that will come to be called romance, and they will use their brains to write paeans of praise to this romance so that their intelligence will fake them out even further until they are unable to distinguish intimacy from dependency."

"It sounds good," said the Creator, "but I have one reservation. Suppose a few, just a few, of these creatures do marry into strengths, or worse, after finding out what we have done to them, make efforts to extricate themselves from these dilemmas?"

"Don't worry, Boss," Satan replied. "We're going to create an institution called divorce. If things get so bad that they can't tolerate one another, then they'll be free to separate and make the same mistake all over again with a new partner."

"That's not what I meant," replied the Master of the Universe. "Suppose some of these creatures decide to do something about their condition. Suppose they decide not to escape, or suppose some learn from their mistakes. They might begin to deal with one another differently, and get some understanding, and perhaps pass that understanding on to others and then produce children whom they teach and rear in these new habits. If such a mutation occurred, the whole thing could lead in no time to some kind of evolutionary process, and who knows where it would all end?"

"We hadn't thought of that. I'll call another meeting of my committee."

Six days went by again, and a new plan was ready. "I think we have solved the problem," reported Satan. "You were absolutely right. We did some projections on the future course of things, and, just as you suggested, that kind of evolutionary process nullifying the curse would have occurred and spread as rapidly as a plague, somewhere around the end of the nineteenth century. But we have found a way that is guaranteed to retard such a growth process; and the beautiful part is that, just like the curse, it will be nourished by human strengths rather than countered by them. Like the curse, it will join that side of being human that denies life's biological origins, the secret connection that unifies creation. Instead it will continue the curse's success in perverting humanity's most distinguishing characteristic, its intelligence, against itself. We've got it programmed to appear at just the right time, too, the early part of the twentieth century."

"Wonderful!" exclaimed the Lord of Hosts. "What will it be called?"

"Well," asked the Devil, "how about psychotherapy?"

Interlude

≈ ≈ ≈ ≈ ≈

Myths are lies that lead to the truth
PICASSO

FAUST: What are you thinking about?
OEDIPUS: The usual, my fate.
FAUST: Don't you ever stop?
OEDIPUS: It's very difficult. Sometimes I succeed for a
    while, but then someone writes another book about
    my meaning and I have to start over.
FAUST: Well, I don't know how you do it. If they paid
    that much attention to me I'd never have time to
    read. I have all I can do to keep up as it is.
OEDIPUS: What's behind *your* obsession?
FAUST: I have no choice. I made a compact with Satan,

remember. My soul for knowledge. How did I know there would ever be that much knowledge? I'm on a treadmill. Every time I think I'm caught up, I've fallen behind. Have you any idea how many books are finished every day or how much research is started every week? It's absolutely devilish.

OEDIPUS: I have the opposite problem. So much is written about me I never get the chance to lust after anything else. I'm totally focused on myself. Have you any idea what it's like to be in analysis for 2,500 years? And it's not like I get a month off in the summer.

FAUST: Well, at least you must have worked a lot of things out.

OEDIPUS: Are you kidding? I'm still impotent.

FAUST: Actually, something similar has happened to me. I thought knowledge was power; it seems more like quicksand.

OEDIPUS: I know the feeling, stuck and sinking.

FAUST: Say, speaking of all that analysis, I've read what everyone's written about you, of course, but I always wondered. I mean . . . no one ever seemed to ask . . . but . . . well . . . what was it like with her?

OEDIPUS: What do you mean?

FAUST: You know . . . with your mother.

OEDIPUS: No one ever did ask me that.

FAUST: I'm basically curious; any knowledge interests me.

OEDIPUS: Well, if you want to know the truth . . .

FAUST: Yes?

OEDIPUS: It never happened.

FAUST: Come on, what are you saying?

OEDIPUS: The whole thing was supposed to be a joke.

When we first started rehearsing we could hardly get our lines out; we were rolling all over the stage. It was supposed to be a melodrama, satire . . .

FAUST: . . . and the world took it seriously by mistake?

OEDIPUS: Sophocles became jealous of all the kudos Aristophanes was receiving for his comedies. He thought he'd try his hand at comedy, also. That's why he came up with something really ludicrous. After all, sex with your mother! And that moment when I rip my eyes out, we thought everyone would howl . . . instead they tried to find meaning in the act.

FAUST: And you've never been able to live it down?

OEDIPUS: You may be chained to the treadmill of your fate, but at least it's real.

FAUST: In one way it isn't.

OEDIPUS: How's that?

FAUST: I hate opera.

OEDIPUS: I can see where that could be a problem.

FAUST: Isn't it remarkable how we never change?

OEDIPUS: Nor seem to help others change much either. But you have to admit that I touch the human soul more deeply. Sophocles may not have realized what he was doing, but I have survived because my story got to the formative matrix of human existence.

FAUST: Rubbish! It astounds me that I have to remind you about your origins. Nothing could have been further from the Greek mind than unconscious sexual fantasies. Their concern was *hubris*, pride. The important issue was their relationship with the gods, not with their parents; it was their struggle with fate; their conflict with the cosmic forces of determinism and free will . . . to use the

rubrics of my metaphor, Sophocles was concerned
with salvation.

OEDIPUS: But are not fate, determinism, free will, salvation the issues that underlie all therapy?

FAUST: Yes and no. They are the issues that underlie all
human encounter, so naturally they are implicit in
all human efforts to bring change. But the trans-
forming power that those ideas have in the drama
of the human soul is often lost in that technocracy
you call therapy.

OEDIPUS: Well, for my part, I have been eternally grate-
ful to Freud for resurrecting me from my stodgy
classicism by showing everyone the universality of
my being.

FAUST: This may shock you, but I, for one, do not believe your story has survived because you touch
something deep in the human spirit. On the contrary, I think your popularity is due to the fact
that you are a convenient displacement. By fo-
cusing on you, people don't have to focus
on me.

OEDIPUS: How can you say that? My name has become
synonymous with the struggle for self-awareness.

FAUST: *I am the important myth of civilization* that nobody
wants to face. The essential question of human
existence is not how your family did you in; it's
maintaining your integrity. The struggle to preserve your own being is far more important than
the issues of how you got to be the way you are.
No, the reason you are popular is *not* because you
are essential, but because so long as people are
fascinated by your story they don't have to be re-
minded of *mine*. You've become an escape, and
therapy, far from being a force for change let alone

a path to salvation, is turning into civilization's mechanism of defense.

OEDIPUS: That's what I get for engaging with a medieval mind—scholasticism and specious reasoning. How much salvation has all your studying gotten you? Frankly, one of the factors that has diluted the power originally inherent in my struggle is the present obsession with information. What you said about the publishing of books and research is nowhere more true than in the disciplines of the helping professions.

FAUST: Mephistopheles has seduced them, too?

OEDIPUS: Sometimes it does seem Satanic. Do you have any idea how many behavior patterns now have names, how many idiosyncracies have labels, how many foibles are called symptoms, how many approaches there are to change, how many factors can be blamed for no change? In the good old days everyone recognized that the key to change was the therapeutic relationship. Today, under the guise of trying to be more sophisticated, they've encrusted the basic tool with coating upon coating of irrelevancies. The therapist of today is not more knowledgeable, merely more confused. And the pursuit of data has become a form of substance abuse. Professionals ingest it to calm their anxiety; only they reach a threshold very quickly and constantly are on the lookout for more powerful stuff.

FAUST: You mean they've mistaken complexity for depth.

OEDIPUS: I always thought you equated knowledge with power.

FAUST: Don't you understand? It didn't work. My learning never transformed me, because I gave up my integrity to obtain it. Simply put, integrity is not

a function of information. You believe you can
control your destiny by looking inward; I believe,
or used to believe, control came from looking beyond ourselves. What I have really learned, the
bottom line, is that the problem of destiny has
nothing to do with either kind of learning.

OEDIPUS: With what then?

FAUST: With our commitments. With what we believe,
with what we treasure most, with what we would
give our lives for, with what we would sell our
souls for.

OEDIPUS: But most people don't know what that is.

FAUST: Exactly, and whenever that's the case looking at
one's past makes little difference. If you want people to influence their own destiny, they must know
what they believe.

OEDIPUS: But what about the divorce rate, the increase
in homosexuality, anorexia, abuse, and the problems of single-parent families, two-income families, and so on?

FAUST: You're not going to like this, but from my perspective most family problems are fads, just like
their cures. Anorexia will go the way of TB. Abuse
will go off stage like influenza. And for eons divorce rates will fluctuate like the levels of the sea
and gender issues will become prominent and re-
cede like the polar caps. The problem is no one
lives long enough to see these things recycle. They
usually come up only once in a mature person's
lifetime, so with a few exceptions there's no one
around who is vigorous enough or who still cares
enough to point out that we've been through all
this before. Besides, they don't always emerge in
the same form, so it's easy to miss the similarity,

as in the way the carcinogen has replaced the communist as society's focus of anxiety. These things don't get cured; they simply go away.

OEDIPUS: Your cynical aloofness startles me. I begin to see why you were capable of making a pact with the Devil.

FAUST: I always know I've made a good point when someone begins to diagnose me.

OEDIPUS: But if we take your position that learning is not the answer and if your also say that looking inward is not the answer, then how do we make progress at all?

FAUST: Well, I, for one, have decided to switch rather than fight.

OEDIPUS: You're going to become a consultant?

FAUST: No, a publisher. As long as Mephistopheles is going to seduce everyone into reading all the time, I might as well get something out of it. We've made a new pact. I keep telling everyone that destiny is a function of information, and he gets authors to write books. We've already created a book club. The Disease of the Month.

OEDIPUS: You're gonna sell a lot of books.

FAUST: We think so.

OEDIPUS: I have to admit some degree of sympathy for your position, but I can't be content with ridicule. I think people can simply not understand their fate, not know how to get unstuck. Though I have to add I don't have a way out for them either.

[At this point both men became silent. Then they became aware of the presence of a third figure appearing out of the mist.]

CASSANDRA: Good evening, gentlemen. Any new ideas about salvation?

OEDIPUS: How did you know we were discussing that?

CASSANDRA: One doesn't have to be a prophet to make that guess.

FAUST: We've been at it for hours, but we seem to have gone nowhere, come full circle, actually.

CASSANDRA: But that's been happening for centuries. Besides, that's your fate Faust, and your destiny Oedipus, never really to know.

FAUST: And I suppose you've made progress in understanding the human condition?

CASSANDRA: Actually, I think at last I have. It doesn't matter, of course, no one ever believes what I say, anyway.

OEDIPUS: Try us—that only happens in the world of reality; here among us myths it's different.

CASSANDRA: I doubt that, but as long as you asked for it. I overheard you both talking on my way over. The dilemma was the same in my time. The disease was not isolated in the House of Atreus; it was rampant among all the Greeks, and it has been passed down generation to generation like some cellular process to all families ever since.

OEDIPUS: You are, of course, talking about *pride*.

CASSANDRA: No, I am talking about *certainty!* It is our undying quest for *certainty* and the resulting reductionism which inevitably follows that allows the Furies to spin out our fate.

FAUST: Then you agree with me about the folly of learning.

CASSANDRA: It is not a matter of knowledge or no knowledge but which knowledge.

OEDIPUS: You're with me, then; the knowledge that's important is insight.

CASSANDRA: What I have to say is neither for nor against learning, nor does it take sides in the dispute between self-knowlege and worldly knowledge. Those are your divisions, not mine.

OEDIPUS: Go on.

CASSANDRA: For me it all began with the battle for my birthplace, Troy. For nearly three millenia years poets and historians have focused on that polarization between Greeks and Trojans, caught up in the romance of that whore Helen. (It wasn't her face that launched a thousand ships.) But I obtained a different perspective on things; for I was the only one who was intimate with both cities, starting out as the daughter of Priam, my country's king, and dying as the lover of Agamemnon, my father's enemy. I was thus the only one who saw that beyond the specious differences was a terrifying similarity. The differences between my beloved Troy and hated Argos did not matter. They were different nations, yes, in different locations, yes, with different rulers, yes. But the denial was absolutely the same.

OEDIPUS: Freud always said you begin by analyzing the resistances, not by immediately offering new insight.

CASSANDRA: Talk about resistance!

OEDIPUS: I'm sorry; you're right; go on.

CASSANDRA: I thought a great deal about all that denial and wondered how the gods could be so sure that my curse—never to be able to pierce its veil—would last, throughout the centuries it turns out. Surely someone, some group, some school of thought would face reality some time. Then, one day I realized my mistake. I was denying the denial. I was seeing it as a weakness, as an effort to avoid reality. Phrasing the problem that way was precisely what the gods wanted; it formatted the question in such a way that the truth could never be revealed. The real molder of denial, I came to see, was not the absence of something, such as courage, but the presence of something, the pursuit of certainty to be exact. You see, if the gods had merely set us up with a bad habit, the habit eventually might have changed, but being gods they knew better, so they made sure to substitute a seductive habit instead. We avoid the truth about our personal destinies not because no one wants to face them; on the contrary, everyone is dying to find out. But we pursue it in a way that prevents us from accepting responsibility for our fate. In short, civilization is not the result of repression; rather it takes shape out of the manifestations of denial.

FAUST: Reminds me of the spells they conjured up in my time.

CASSANDRA: But the crucial point is this: The reason people have no power over these forces they are obsessed with understanding is not because they are too strong, or too mysterious, or too hidden, or too ubiquitous for that matter, but because they actually do not exist . . . well, that's not quite right, they do exist; but they are really quite irrelevant to our destiny.

FAUST: You're mocking all the academic traditions of Western civilization.

CASSANDRA: Only the Northeast-Interlocking-Intellectual-Directorate. The quest for certainty has produced a fascination with reducing everything to its basic components; everything must have an answer. Only the poets are unafraid of ambiguity. Everyone else goes to experts. It is true that in my day we sought oracles, but today people still want the oracular, whether from their therapist, their physician, their minister, or their politician. The helping professions have been turned into certaintizers. At least in my day at Delphi they had the good sense not to be too specific.

OEDIPUS: They had to be ambiguous; they didn't know what experts know today.

CASSANDRA: Well, what do they know today? No more than they knew then.

FAUST: I completely agree with you there. It does not seem to occur to anyone that if ancient literature makes sense today, then the forces that mold our lives have not really changed.

CASSANDRA: But it is not only those forces that have remained the same, so it is with our way of thinking about them. In my day fate was attributed to the gods; we could not risk the idea that circumstance was dumb and that destiny depends more on our personal response to challenge. So we had a god for every dimension of existence or the environment: love, war, sleep, the sea, the earth, the sky, time itself. And we gave our fate over into their imaginary hands rather than take responsibility for the fact that the hostility of most environments depends less on the toxic elements within them than on the response of the organism to challenge.

FAUST: But surely people no longer worship those icons. They have become more sophisticated.

CASSANDRA: Not so. The Pantheon is still there, disguised by what you call sophistication. It is true no one worships Demeter or Neptune any longer, nor calls upon Aphrodite or Mars in his greatest despair, but the pantheon of outside forces to which mortals attribute their personal destiny is as present as before; the gods have merely changed their names. Now they are known as *genes, gender, class, race, symptoms, the age, peer groups, statistics* (which doubles as a Trojan Horse) and Zeus, all-powerful king of the gods, is now called *a dysfunctional family of origin.* I think it was Euripides, my countryman, who caught it best. How did he put it? Oh, yes, "we are continually molding our character and calling it fate."

FAUST: That's pretty heavy, Cassy, but why do you have to be so pessimistic?

CASSANDRA: Isn't it remarkable how all I ever wanted to do was speak the truth, and my name has become synonymous with pessimism? At least with the old Pantheon there was humor, and it produced art that enabled humans to look at themselves from outside themselves. Besides, not everyone believed in the gods, and playwrights were allowed to make fun of them. But who dares satirize these deities of certainty today?

OEDIPUS: You know, you're making it very difficult to distinguish the quest for certainty from schizophrenia.

CASSANDRA: At last. You're getting it. You see my concern is with the human spirit. Not the male spirit, or the female spirit, not the black spirit nor the white spirit. And the liberation of the spirit always comes from a direction that moves toward understanding the unity of life, not from the dichotomizing, bifurcating, reductionizing, certaintizing forces of anxiety that polarize and squeeze our thoughts into all-or-nothing categories. The materialism inherent in idolatry lies not in the objects of its adoration but in the effect of what that adoration denies.

FAUST: But, Cassandra, the same thinking that you call reductionistic has led to powerful political forces that have brought great improvement of the human lot and the lifting of many human spirits.

CASSANDRA: Do you think I am opposed to equality for women, or homes for the homeless, or guidance for children? But improvements in society do not automatically bring change in the human soul. I do not believe the salvation of humanity can be reduced to issues of justice and gender. Causes are notorious for the way they allow their champions to deny responsibility for their own personal destiny. Spirituality is not implanted; it is freed. Salvation depends on struggling for clarity, not certainty, and that means *preserving* the ambiguity of the human condition and the perplexing paradoxes of protoplasm. I would have people ask questions like:

- How does love trigger the disintegration of the loved one?
- How do efforts to control another become an adaptation to the other's weakness?
- Why does dependency kill?
- How does rigidity in one person create self-doubt in another?
- Why is it the nature of craziness to drive those who try to understand it in others crazy?

- How does support weaken? or challenge become a form of caring?
- When does responsibility for others become irresponsible?
- How do words lose their power when they are used to overpower

These are the essential questions for the future of human destiny. But don't worry; no one ever believes me.

FAUST: If I understand you, Cassandra, what you are saying is that the evolution of humanity depends less on technological, administrative, and managerial changes than on changing the way we conceptualize our problems.

CASSANDRA. Precisely.

OEDIPUS: But that would require changing our myths.

CASSANDRA: You hit it again.

FAUST: I mean, I would have to assume that the devil is in *me*. And Eddi-pus over there, he'd have to put his eyes back into his head. I don't know how I'd live with myself . . . on the other hand, if it would stop all that singing . . .

[Suddenly, Oedipus bolts]

FAUST: Where are you going? Aren't you with us?

OEDIPUS: Yes, yes, I agree, but it's Sunday.

FAUST: What's that got to do with anything?

OEDIPUS: It will soon be noon.

FAUST: So?

OEDIPUS: Well, my God, I forgot to call my mother.

BONDS
AND
BINDS

There is a curious connection between the way people think and the way people bond. To the extent they tend to frame life's issues in black-and-white, either/or, on-and-off alternatives, to that extent their responses to the challenges of life will lack resiliency. And the more likely it is that their bonds will become binds. On the other hand, to the extent individuals are unafraid of ambiguity and can even come to appreciate its value, then the repertoire of their relational responses is broadened, and that in turn will enrich the alternatives in their style of thinking.

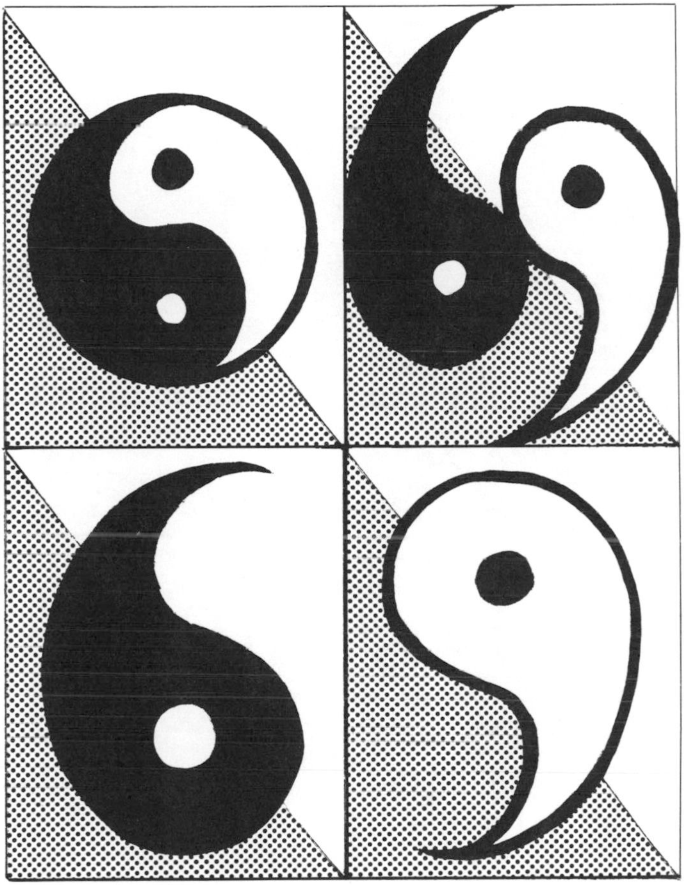

Symbiosis

"I want you out," said the Bacterium to its Virus.

"What are you talking about?" the Virus responded.

"Out," repeated the Bacterium, "out of my space."

"All the way?"

"Beyond my limits," said the Bacterium.

"Why?" asked the Virus.

"I no longer want to share my existence with you."

"Things don't happen that way."

"I know," said the Bacterium.

"We've lived together a long time," the Virus added.

"Nonetheless," said the Bacterium, "it's my space and I no longer want to share it with you."

"You don't know what you are doing," responded the Virus.

"I was never more determined."

"But after all this time?"

"I want to be myself," answered the Bacterium.

"But you can't be without me."

"I can't be because of you."

"You are going against your nature," said the Virus.

"Only against my past behavior."

"What's the difference?"

"That's what I want to find out."

"You're considering a different Virus, then?" asked the Virus.

"Not right now," said the Bacterium.

"You would try it on your own?"

"At the beginning, anyway."

"I've done my best. I was always benign."

"It has to do with me, not with you."

"But what were you before I came along?"

"Much the same as I am now."

"Before we came together you weren't near what you are now."

"That's not what I meant," said the Bacterium.

"I don't understand."

"I haven't really changed."

"But you have, greatly."

"No, I still depend on you in order to be me."

"What's wrong with that?"

"That's transformation, not change."

"What's the difference?"

"In change, something remains the same."
"I made you you," said the Virus.
"You helped greatly."
"Helped? We need one another."
"We don't actually know that."
"How could you doubt it?"
"It's just a new thought."
"We became one organism," said the Virus.
"That's why I want you out," responded the Bacterium.
"You'll regress."
"For a while."
"For a while? Forever."
"I am determined."
"How will you function without me?" asked the Virus.
"I no longer need you to turn me on."

V: It's not fair.
B: It's vital.
V: What will I do?
B: Find another host.
V: Suppose they're all occupied?
B: New ones come along all the time.
V: Suppose they're not compatible?
B: That's not my problem.
V: I really have turned you off.
B: No, I turned me off.
V: Suppose you turned me off?
B: What's the difference?
V: We're that close?

B: Till now, inseparable.
V: There is a difference.
B: What's that?
V: Whether or not you've really changed.
B: How could you doubt it?
V: It depends on the turn-off.
B: This time I controlled the switch.
V: Maybe it was only a switch.
B: What's your point?
V: Who did you turn off?
B: I won't let you affect me.
V: You're avoiding my question.
B: I am trying to define myself.
V: By turning me off?
B: No, by turning me off to you.
V: I affect you that much?
B: Automatically.
V: Then you haven't changed.
B: You no longer control me.
V: It's my presence, isn't it?

I'm set to go.
Goodbye.
Still determined?
Definitely.
I have one more question.
What?
Why didn't you leave?
I'm not in your space.

Does that really matter?
It's the basic issue.
From your perspective.
What do you mean by that?
You adapted as much as I.
But you were the invasive one.
You gave me the opening.
I couldn't help myself.
You didn't allow others in.
I was particularly sensitive to you.
Because of my makeup or yours?
It doesn't matter now.
In one way it does.
How's that?
Survival.
That's why I must separate.
I was becoming malignant?
Yes.
Because of my makeup or yours?
I just got used to you.
You are understating compatibility.
Please leave.
Is there no way we can live together?
Only if you stay outside.
You'll want me back.
Only if you stay outside.
Then what's the use?
Something might evolve.

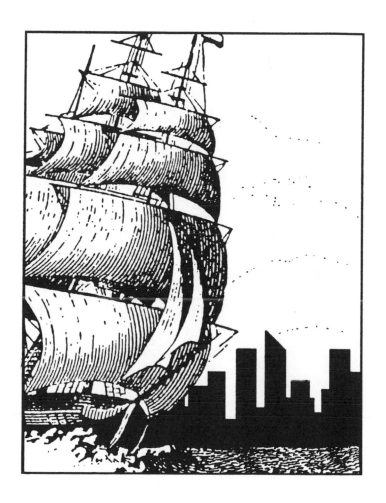

Attachment

Once upon a time, a storm-tossed ship gave up one of its passengers. He clung to debris that had gone over the side with him and floated for a few hours. Finally, he could hold on no longer, and he let go.

When he came to, he found himself on an uncharted island. The island was perfect. Tall palms, verdant brush, sparkling hills. Hardly believing it was real, he tried to wake himself from his dream, though with some fear that if he succeeded, he would find himself dead. It appeared, however, that he was very much alive. Curiosity and hunger moved him to explore.

As he invaded the jungle's depths, he was struck by the calm. There were no loud cries of birds or beasts, and there seemed to be, if anything, a certain order everywhere.

He spent most of that first day feasting with his eyes and mouth. Many delicious fruits and nuts were easily available to his reach, and his stomach was soon satisfied. But so wondrous were the colors, the more his eyes took in, the more he wanted to devour. As the first evening came on, and he prepared for sleep, he found that the climate, while cool, was in no way chilling. Wearily he lay down to bed upon a mattress of soft leaves, thankful to be still alive, yet a little scared at being so alone.

When he woke the next morning, he was no longer by himself. Sitting all about him in a circle were men, women, and children. Some of the most beautiful men, women, and children he had ever seen. They had taken care not to awaken him, and they had brought gifts. Did they think he was a god? As he bestirred himself, they came over, offering food and drink. One who seemed to be a leader appeared to be asking if he were ill or hurt. He did not speak their language, but they easily understood his gestures. He quickly discovered that theirs, too, were easily understandable.

Indeed, he found that everything about these people was simple and graceful. They accepted him immediately and made him one of them. He learned their ways of communication.

But there was one idea he was totally unable to convey, that at times he wanted to be by himself. On this island, no one was ever left alone. When a baby was born, the people did not sever the umbilical cord. The child thus remained extremely close to its mother throughout its infancy. If the mother wanted to have another child, the umbilical cord was severed, but only from the mother, and her end was then reattached by a simple surgical procedure to one of the older women, who continued to care for the child until it was ready to mate. As part of the wedding ceremony, the future partners' cords were severed, but again, only the ends that were connected to the parent surrogates, and, as each loose end was attached to the intended spouse, the bride and groom were thus united. In those cases where a mother had had only one child, the cord was reattached directly from natural mother to spouse.

Shortly before a wife was to give birth, the husband and wife had their cords unjoined and the husband could then become attached to another female ready to leave her mother or mother surrogate. He also had the option of rejoining with his own mother, if she had not rejoined with her husband, or he could join again with some mother surrogate, perhaps his original one.

While to our modern sense, this way of bonding might seem primitive, even uncivilized, the effects of this constant attachment on society were astounding. Anger was unknown, depression was easily cured, crime was unheard of, envy and jealousy never spawned, and competition and rivalry were totally absent. There was no such thing as embarrassment, nor any of those behavior patterns that we have come to call neuroses. If there was fear or anxiety, it was experienced only during that period of time when someone accidentally "lost" a partner. Such loss was always replaced as soon as possible, however, and the anxiety would quickly subside. Indeed, it was probably only because the islanders remembered these instances of loss that some sense of aloneness was known at all. Despite this, the expected death of a family member never increased anxiety greatly, because everyone had the assurance that the family would quickly make a replacement available. Such back-up also may have meant that individuals were freer to die.

The man spent many years on the island, at one point becoming attached to a woman with whom he found mutual attraction. But he soon realized that he could not suffer her omnipresence, and rather than introduce the spoilation of bickering to these lovely people, he asked for a "separation." There was perhaps one time when he thought he had found a woman who might have tried his way of life, but she changed her mind at the last minute and soon tied the knot with another. As he retold it later, her change of mind seemed to have less to do with any failure of nerve on her part than with a concern to calm her own family. They seemed to be becoming increasingly upset over the prospect of their daughter's living unattached.

After several years, the proverbial ship appeared and he left these wonderful people sadly. As always, he was astounded by their reaction, this time to his departure. For as kind and close as they had seemed, they now appeared to take his loss with perfect equanimity. In fact, he found himself wondering if they had ever cared at all. Whereas he, though he had been unable to be totally a part of their life, now found himself almost totally unable to separate.

When he returned home, his family was overjoyed to see him again, though his wife, thinking he had died, had soon remarried. He himself remarried shortly thereafter, and the pain of the loss subsided. He tried to publish an account of his experience in several scholarly journals, but they all said it was too fantastic. He finally sold it as a fantasy. One reviewer thought his style too realistic.

Many years later, a ship traveling in the same waters happened upon a gloriously beautiful, uncharted island. A crew went forth to explore. They were met by a patrol who ushered them firmly to headquarters. When it was seen that the men meant no harm, they were freed, and their ship was allowed to come into the port of the island's bustling metropolis. The men were quite surprised to see such an advanced society so far removed from the rest of civilization. Newspapers contained all the sections of any modern daily: current events, crime, economic issues, sports fashions, the usual range of advertisement.

"You know," said one of the crew, "as a child, I once heard a story about a beautiful island just like this. A man claimed to have lived there for several years. He described it as one of the loveliest places he had ever seen, with the kindest and warmest people. In many ways he could have been describing this very place. Except that he said it was very primitive, and there was one other thing also. he said, "If you could feature this, everyone went around constantly tied to someone else by their umbilical cords."

"Oh, I remember him," the tour guide said, as he ushered them all into a waiting hovercraft. "That's just the way it used to be here," he continued, straining above the noise of the motors as they exploded into full throttle. "But after he left," the pilot shouted back through the spray, "we all cut them off."

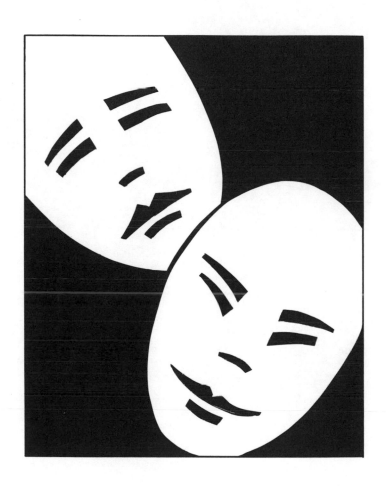

Jean and Jane

Jean and Jane were very good friends. But Jean and Jane were in no way alike. For Jane was very friendly, always cheerful, always happy. But Jean was more reflective, rarely laughing, rarely smiling.

While Jean stayed pretty much to herself, even in groups, Jane was the life of every party. While Jane entered any room and immediately attracted a crowd, Jean entered any room and remained so inconspicuous it was as if she were not there.

Jean was not really less attractive, yet she attracted less. Jane was not really a superficial butterfly, yet she was never alone.

As time went on Jean began to worry about the

difference. "Why it it," she thought, "that Jane always has more fun? Why is it that I, on the other hand, am always so unhappy? Does Jane simply know better how to win friends and influence people? If so, where did she learn it, and why haven't I, Jean, learned it?" Jean reflected on her own patterns and came to see that there was no clear reason for their difference.

She and Jane were the same age, had about the same physical attributes. Ok, Jane was a blonde. But some men liked brunettes. They each could sing; each played about the same game of tennis. Ok, Jane was a better swimmer, but she couldn't play golf!

The more Jean thought about Jane, the more depressed she became. It was not just envy. Jane was the reflection of her, Jean's, own potential. Jane, right now, in the present, was all that Jean ever wanted to be but somehow found herself unable to be. As Jean brooded about this problem, things worsened. She isolated herself more. Then she functioned less. Eventually she stopped going out at all. And who would have wanted to be around her anyway?

Throughout this time, Jane continued on her way. Almost every evening the phone rang. At the club she was invited to every activity. For she was, after all, a pleasure to be with. Even at work others admitted that they worked harder in her presence, and she almost never had to eat by herself.

Finally, Jean, with great effort, managed to establish a relationship—with a therapist. Weekly she went, and she began to discuss her problem, how no one seemed to want her, how she was usually left out of things, if not completely ignored, how jealous she was of Jane.

Slowly, she talked about her own behavior. Carefully, she revealed her inner feelings. Hesitantly, she discussed her past.

As time went by, she made some progress, but it always seemed to be overshadowed by Jane, who, if this was possible, became even more popular than before. Thus Jane continued to be a reminder to Jean of what a woman could be. "Hah," thought Jean one day, about 6 months after she had begun to work on her problem, "why, if Jane ever had to see someone for professional help, she'd probably be through in a matter of weeks."

It was in the midst of one of these doldrums that Jean, upon entering her therapist's office, was astounded to see Jane coming out.

"Hi, Jean," said Jane in her usual cheery way.

"Hi," responded Jean, surprised.

"What are you doing here?" asked Jane sweetly.

"Me?" said Jean. "Why I've been coming here for almost a year. This is my regular weekly appointment. What brings you here today?"

"Well, we had to switch today. I've been seeing the doctor for several years now," said Jane, still her usual eager self. "I wish I could cut down to only once a week."

"But how often do you come?" inquired Jean, incredulously.

"Usually three times, but sometimes if I'm really desperate he fits me in for a fourth."

"Desperate!" exclaimed Jean.

"Oh, yes," responded Jane. "You know, Jean, I can't tell you how surprised I am to find you here. You always seemed so sure of yourself. You're always so self-reliant, always so able to be alone. You have no idea how

I admire your independence, your tolerance for solitude, your capacity to keep your distance."

Jean was still trying to come from behind the other side of the mirror as she finally asked, "But, Jane, what's your problem?"

"You mean, you can't tell?" chirped Jane. "I am totally unable to say no."

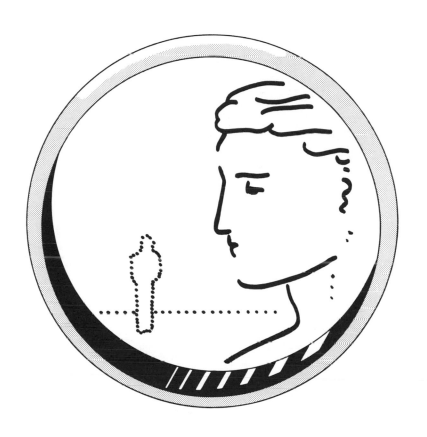

The Magic Ring

Once upon a time there was an alluring woman who had everything she wanted. She was married to a handsome and intelligent man who made a very successful living. They had much in common, including two children who were both bright and talented, and her husband gave her freedom to spend her days as she wished. She had little to complain about, past or present.

Then one day her husband suddenly, and without any preparation, left her for another woman. The shock, the surprise, and the shattering of her world were complete, and it took a long time for her to recover. As she did, she began to worry. If it could happen once, it could happen again, and she never wanted to endure that experience again.

How could she live among men, for she did like their companionship, and not endanger herself? This question she pondered for some time, but all those she asked admitted they had no answer. If anything, they seemed to fear it could happen to them.

At last she asked her saintly grandmother, who had lost her husband many years ago and never sought another.

"Ah," said her grandmother, "I know well how you feel and I am going to help you. As you know, when your grandfather died suddenly I, too, was disconsolate. He had been my whole life. I had withheld nothing. When he left so unexpectedly, I wondered how I could go on; in fact, I really didn't want to, but as luck would have it, I was given something by my grandmother that has protected me ever since."

"What was that?" the young woman asked.

"Come here, my child," she said. "You see this ring?"

"Yes, grandmother," the woman answered, "as long as I have known you, I have always seen you wear it."

"Right, my child, and I have never taken it off. This is no ordinary ring," she continued. "It is a magic ring, and I am going to give it to you, for I am so old that I do not need its protection any longer."

"But how does it protect?" the woman asked.

"This ring has great power," the saintly grandmother replied, "and it will protect you in two ways. First, it will enable you to keep your feelings in check. No matter how attractive any man is, you may feel free to be as close to him as you wish, knowing that just when your own level of involvement reaches a critical stage, your feelings will automatically shut off. You may not yourself understand what is happening. You may think you actually no longer like the man. You may even begin to find fault with him or appear to discover a less attractive side. That is not important. What is important is that you can feel totally free to be with as many men as you wish and get as close, or be as attractive, as you desire. For no matter how the man desires you, you will never lose yourself in love."

"But, grandmother," said the woman, "I think I would really like to love again, without limit; it's just that I'm so afraid."

"I understand," answered the elder, "but you must let me finish, for I have not yet explained the other power in this ring."

She paused and slipped the ring off her finger, polished it a bit, and took her granddaughter's hand. Then she continued, "As I said, the ring has another power. Besides turning your feelings off when they reach a crucial stage, the ring will enable you to know immediately if a man is himself afraid of involvement, or, for some reason, unable to become involved. With such knowledge you will be able to choose those men with whom you can let yourself go completely, totally without risk."

"Oh, grandmother," cried the woman, "how wonderful!"

She took the magic ring, kissed it, and placed it on her finger.

"I shall never take it off again," she said, "never . . . until I am as old as you."

"I am glad to hear you say that," said the old woman, "for this ring is of no use to those who are wishy-washy in their commitment. You must never again go anywhere without it, not even for a minute, lest you be snared unawares."

"I promise," she said enthusiastically and went forth to her newfound freedom.

For years she dated men of all ages and description, rich and poor, handsome and intelligent, athletes and aesthetes. With risk no longer a factor, she could be as adorable as she wished, and when some men did indeed come to adore her, she easily found a way to cast them aside, thus making room for others. When, on the other hand, she wished to let her own feelings go without limit, she naturally, almost by instinct, chose only those unable to fall in love with her, either by nature (homosexuals, for example) or by situation (happily married men who wanted a pretty woman by their side).

And, she never, never, ever went anywhere without her magic ring.

As time went by, she realized that without the worry of risk she was able to cultivate her charm, thus making herself even more attractive. Her air of abandonment drew men like half-blind moths to some far-off flickering light, which, since it was not really burning, produced more disappointment than destruction. For they flew in, hardly in control, only to bounce off something hard, whereupon, half-stunned, they fluttered a bit but then flew on toward other attractions.

Almost oblivious to how it worked, she continued to allow herself to burn with desire only for her minister, her doctor, her supervisors, or those colleagues at work who, her magic ring told her, as if by instinct, were absolutely safe.

One day, as she was about to be picked up for

lunch by a man from one of these categories—one about whom she felt safest, and therefore, one whom she had permitted into her most delicious fantasies—she rushed to meet him without her ring. Realizing what she had done, she started back, just as he drove up.

"Come on," he beckoned. "Sorry I'm late."

Caught short, she reassured herself. "This is ridiculous. I already know about him. I'll just make sure not to meet anyone else today."

As she slipped into her car beside him, he was rolling down his window. Then she saw him toss something out onto the pavement.

"What was that?" she asked, settling down.

"Oh, nothing," he answered, smiling, "just some stupid ring my saintly grandmother gave me many years ago."

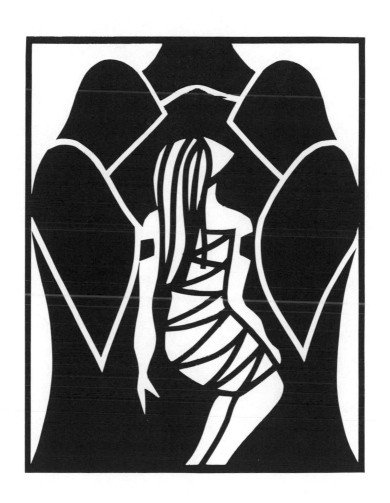

The Lesson

At 5:00 A.M. on a cold, damp morning, three figures, hooded, silent, with a single purpose in mind, stole quickly, carefully up the stairway of a sleep-filled home and, after toeing their way adroitly to one of the bedrooms on the second floor, burst in on its inhabitant. Surrounding her bed, in the choreography of their intent, they simultaneously lunged toward the sleeping figure, who barely struggled, so taken was she by surprise. Binding her in her own bedsheets, they carried her down to the street again, and as two bent her arms behind her back, the third began to slam his fists into her wriggling, writhing body.

"How dare you," he said venomously as his left hand made contact with her ribs.

"Just who do you think you are?" he added, his teeth gritting together. "Did you really think we'd let you get away with this?" he added, and back slapped her across the face. It was only the tips of his fingers that made contact, but the effect was all the more stinging because of the whip-like path of his arc.

She tried to duck his onslaught but could not, so rigidly was she held in place by the other two.

"Who gave you the right to go off on your own?" her tormentor questioned. He was breathing heavily now.

"Selfish bitch." This time when he clenched his fist, he kept his pointer finger out and poked her in the side. The quickness of her body's withdrawal invited him further, and he poked her again.

She hung there in the others' arms, confused. She had been sleeping deeply when they seized her. Now all responses were totally automatic. It seemed as though she had barely shaken the drowsiness from her mind when she was about to collapse into unconsciousness again. She tried to understand what was happening. She heard his comments, his questions. She could feel his breathing, but she was unable to respond.

And the other two offered nothing.

"You think you're special, don't you?" she heard, but before her mind could form a response, his fist crashed into her lower abdomen, causing her to gasp for air. All her energy went into regulating her breathing again.

"What made you think you don't have to follow the rules?" This time, the question was followed by a numbing sensation across her lips, and she began to sense her warm, viscous blood as it pooled inside her mouth and trickled down the side of her chin.

And the other two offered nothing.

She was sobbing, her torso heaving, as various parts of her body sent competing pain signals to her brain for the right to be recognized. The surprise was gone now. Her wonderment had been preempted by her predicament. She struggled to be free, but there was no escape.

"This will teach you to do as we say," her assailant said through clenched teeth, jerking her head to the side by the ends of her hair. He was nose to nose, his eyes open wide. She kept hers closed, since she could not avoid his gaze, and began to beg for mercy. But something deep within stopped her plea.

"This is what we do to people who think only about themselves," he said authoritatively. "We warned you before, but you did not listen. Now you will receive a lesson you will never forget."

As if on signal, the other two tensed their muscles to hold her even more firmly than before, and he began attacking her ferociously, directing his pain administration to different parts of her body with various methods and techniques: punching, slapping, poking, pinching.

"Please, stop," she was finally able to scream.

But soon she was no longer conscious. She could not hear him, and her pain also had ceased to be a stimulus. So he stopped. It was over—for this time, anyway.

His arms tired, and his body weary of its feral orgy, her husband turned and went back to bed, while her parents let her slip limply to the ground and wafted back to their graves.

She dreamed again.

At 5:00 A.M. on a cold, damp morning, three figures, hooded, silent, with a single purpose in mind, stole quickly, carefully up the stairway of a sleep-filled home and, after toeing their way adroitly to one of the bedrooms on the second floor, burst in on its inhabitant. Surrounding her bed, in the choreography of their intent, they simultaneously lunged toward the sleeping figure, who barely struggled, so taken was she by surprise. Binding her in her own bedsheets, they carried her firmly down to the street again, and as two bent her arms behind her back, the third began to kiss her sweetly. First on her nose, then on her forehead, and then upon each ear.

He held her face tenderly in his hands and softly touched her lips with his. She could feel his strong body pressing her breasts and then his hands caressing them. She wanted to respond. The core of her being felt irrepressible urges . . . to hold him, to return his kisses, to press her body more fully against his, to embrace him totally, but, as before, the other two firmly pinned her arms behind her back and would not permit the slightest move.

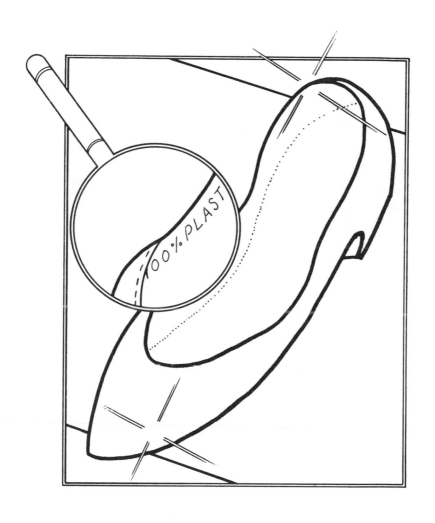

Cinderella

An Address Delivered to the National Association of Family Therapists by Cinderella's Stepmother

Ⅰt is with great apprecia-
tion that I stand here today. On behalf of all the step-
mothers of every age, everywhere, I want to thank you.
Actually, it's hard for me to believe this finally happened. For so many years I wanted the opportunity to
tell my side of the story, but no one would listen. In
truth, no one even thought there was another side.

I am tempted to seize this opportunity to get even,
to rebut and refute all those who have contributed to
branding my stereotype into the world's culture and who
have perpetuated the myth of my meanness. Equal time
is a wonderful elixir. But I fear there is no way I could
do that without appearing defensive. I have decided,
therefore, simply to tell it as it was, or, at least, as it was

according to my perception. You will have to determine the truth. Though, at least, when I am through, I hope it will be from a more evenly weighted point of view.

I first met Cinderella's father at a dance given by the king. It was to celebrate the completion of a new wing of the castle, and Cindy's father had been one of the major contractors. (I should mention, by the way, that we never, never called her Cinderella. She wouldn't hear of it. It wasn't folksy enough.) I had been invited because my dead husband had been one of the original designers. I had just gone through a year of mourning, and this was a kind of coming-out for me. I was struck immediately by the man's gentleness. He had a sadness in his eyes, and somehow his doleful demeanor sparked pity in my heart. He seemed quite intelligent, if quiet, and talked a great deal about his daughter, whom he obviously adored. His wife had died several years previously, and he seemed so choked even to mention it that I never did find out what ailment had done her in. He had lived alone with his teenage daughter, and except for an older, wealthy, widowed sister—about whom I shall have more to say later (the interfering witch)—he had few personal relationships. It was a pleasant enough evening, and I was glad that I had begun to circulate again. I was quite surprised, however, by what was to follow.

For the very next evening he came 'round with a basket of fruit and flowers. My daughters, who both were home that evening, giggled, gasped, and discreetly went out to play. I was overwhelmed. I had never received that much attention from my first husband in all our years together. We went for a walk, talked, and before I knew it, he proposed.

Well, I tried to point out that we hardly knew one

another, but he was very persistent. I told him I needed time to consider it and spent most of the next day plucking daisies. In retrospect, I don't know what was the matter with me. Generally the last thing you would call me is impulsive. But I was lonely. He made a good living that would provide security for my own children, and there was this yearning in me to care for someone. Most of all, maybe I was just plain flattered. Little did I know how soon all that attention would cease. And little did I guess what I was in for with his beloved Cindy.

As soon as we moved in, I went about setting things to rights. While I would not consider myself orderly to a fault, I do believe that order is essential to any fruitful life, though when it comes to kitchens, there I admit to erring on the side of the meticulous.

My daughters, raised in this atmosphere, were naturally tidy, and perhaps it *was* a mistake on my part to expect that Cindy would have exactly the same attitudes. The truth of the matter is that she had none of the same attitudes. She balked immediately at any mention of her assistance in setting the table, fetching water, or cleaning the floor. In fact, I don't think she had ever actually held a broom before.

I tried at first to persuade her that this was important for her own upbringing, as well as for the family, but she would just throw a temper tantrum or run to her father (who always took her side by failing to support me). Often she would go to her room where she seemed to have an infinite capacity for sitting and looking out the window. (And I admit that I was unsure of my own authority—after all, she was not really my daughter.) Sometimes when my own daughters, who were naturally upset at having to do all the work, would taunt her, she would come back with remarks obviously born in those long periods of fantasy. "You just wait and see," she would say. "Some day I won't have to live here any longer. Someday," she would say, "my prince will come."

Things got worse. My daughters became more and more upset about having to do her share of the work, my husband spent more and more time away from the house, and my health, always my best companion, began to leave me. Finally, one day I told Cindy's father that I would have to take my daughters and leave if he was unwilling to support me on this.

That must have gotten to him, because he agreed that Cindy would have to obey me. He was never around, of course, to back me up, but at least it stopped her from running to him whenever she couldn't get her way with me.

So all she did instead was start running to my husband's sister. This sister was, as I said, a wealthy widow with no children of her own and gave Cindy absolutely everything she wanted. This, too, became a problem for my daughters, as she never really accepted them or me. It seemed as though all Cindy would have to do is wish for something, and there was her aunt making it happen.

Once again, things were starting to become intolerable, and that's when this other flake began to show up. He had seen Cindy walking her usual aimless way one day and must have sensed the compatibility immediately. He had nothing to recommend him: no trade, no goals, nor any idea what he would be doing with his life the next hour, let alone the next day. Another dreamer.

And another charmer. Boy, were they made for one another. On the surface so kind and gentle and pleasing, always saying the right thing when they wanted something, and innocent, always so innocent.

He also made passes at my daughters, I should add, but they found him absolutely revolting. Well, one night Cindy and her charming prince just take off and don't come back. At first, I didn't know how they expected to survive (though I have a suspicion that that sister-in-law of mine was in cahoots), and then the most amazing thing comes out. It turns out he really is a prince, the king's only son, of all things. Evidently they had been having a lot of trouble with him. He hadn't been minding his studies, was sneaking certain herbs that are generally forbidden into the castle itself, and had gotten into bad company.

Well, the next thing I hear, Cindy and the prince are getting married in a big, royal affair, the prince has taken to wearing fine clothes and preparing for succession, and everyone is running around saying how Cindy was the best thing that ever happened to him. She sent some servant back to the house for her things, and we never did see her again. You don't think we were invited to the wedding?

I was disappointed, of course, especially for my daughters, but the worst was yet to come. For the palace began to put out this story of the great romance. How the prince had not been seen for a long time because he was actually searching for his one and only, how he had found her in a hovel, and—pardon me, this is the part that really hurts—how she had been almost a slave in her father's house because he had been ensnared by the wiles of this wicked witch.

I don't know how it all got going. Maybe it took off as a natural embellishing of the romance, or maybe it was Cindy's way of getting back at me. In all events, we could not show ourselves in the market for a long time, and finally, to give my daughters a better chance, we moved to another town.

In looking back, however, I don't know if I would have done things differently. I still believe in the values of energy, persistence, and order. Maybe I took on too much responsibility. I should have let her flake out all the way; after all, she was my husband's daughter. Or maybe I should have waited longer 'till I remarried.

One thing I did learn, however. I shouldn't have backed off each time Cindy went to tell her father and aunt how mean I was. I should have gotten "meaner." You know, I think I was the only one who ever took a stand with her. But, given the overall absence of limits, that's the only thing she remembered about me. And maybe, as one of my daughters says, that's why she and her prince persisted in that myth about my meanness. For it was probably the only way they could really live with one another happily ever after.

Reptilian Regressions

Have you ever noticed that while you can make your horse prance and perhaps even your dog dance, you cannot play with your pet alligator, salamander, turtle, or snake? They are deadly serious creatures. It is out of the question to expect them to behave mischievously, let alone irreverently. It is also rare to see them develop a relationship that is nurturing. Playfulness and nurturing appear to have evolved simultaneously, perhaps even as part of one another, and are part of our mammalian heritage. Is it so far-fetched to say, therefore, that in all human communication when we have forgotten "the importance of *not* being earnest," at such moments we have committed a reptilian regression?

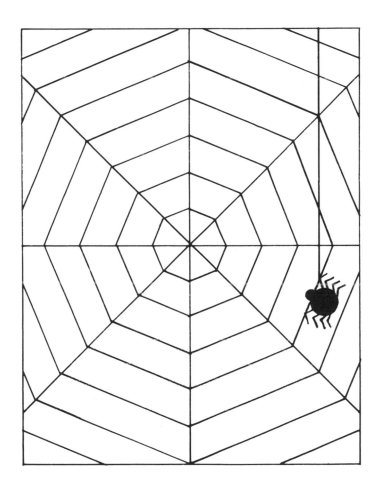

Caught in Her
Own Web

One August evening, as
Mrs. Brown singlehandedly set her household straight,
just outside the kitchen wall, beneath an overhanging
parapet, Ms. Mary Muffet, a spider of the species *Energia
nervosa*, spun a perfect web. Like most other webs of spi-
derdom, it was held together by radiating spokes, each
angling out toward faraway points. But this evening the
angles were all equal. And the distance between the
threads that joined the spokes was also uniform. Ms.
Muffet had produced a set of absolutely regular concen-
tric polygons.

This had never occurred before anywhere in the
entire kingdom of *Arachnid*. Every side of every octagon
was the exact same distance from the one across, whether

measured toward the center or from above. Every strand between was perfectly in line with the next, creating a ladder of parallel steps. No thread slacked anywhere, so that the natural fluorescence designed to attract nourishment glistened with astonishing sparkle. There were no dimming shadows anywhere. The overall effect was of extraordinary delicacy and ominous grace.

Ms. Muffet did not immediately become aware of what she had achieved. As soon as she had finished, she descended quickly, with her usual industry, by spinning a separate dragline, and prepared to wait for the evening's prey in satisfying anticipation for her single-minded labor's reward.

As was her custom, she began to make herself as small as possible, collapsing her legs beneath her body so that she appeared to be little more than a lifeless speck of derelict dirt. Her routine included looking up once to see if there were any glaring irregularities, or, though she would never admit it, if this were her day. She barely glanced. But she saw it: the perfect symmetry. On previous occasions she had had similar starts. But upon closer investigation, she would find some imperfection—a frayed corner perhaps, a slight sag that prevented true parallelism, an uneven spoke that allowed distortion in the wind.

For those who are not familiar with such things, it is not possible to induce symmetry once a web is spun. For such is the nature of webs that whenever one part is realigned, another part will inevitably be thrown off. Were this not the case, spiders would perpetually be producing perfect webs by just spinning in any manner and then going up and fixing the result. The perfect web must be produced on the first try and is as rare as bowling 300, pitching a no-hit game, or opening one's cards to a royal flush. Some say it is most akin to the last. One does not cause these things to happen. They are, rather, the result of what life deals out. Thus most spiders, upon completing their handiwork, do not even bother to check.

Ms. Muffet *always* checked. Whether it was nature or nurture, none of her siblings shared this concern. In fact, as spiderlings much family humor had centered around the improbability of the perfect web. Ms. Muffet, however, always exacting, always precise, always took such comments seriously.

Realizing what might have happened, Ms. Muffet zipped up her elevator thread, examining meticulously every crosshair and bolt. She thought she saw a break, but when she scurried over, she found it was only the play of light. Several more times she nimbly scrambled up the trellis of her dreams, afraid she had spied some imperfection, but each time the defect was not there.

Not wanting to deform her own art in the process of preserving it, Ms. Muffet designed an ingenious scheme for getting close without disturbing the impeccability of her creation. She spun a second web similar in size and in the same plane as the first, not so close that it might be blown into her masterpiece, but near enough that she could clearly see every one of its dimensions. From this scaffolding she continued her search. Up and down she scampered. Now and then she would spin a thread and swing closer, and sometimes she even had the temerity to alight upon The Web itself. But despite the most exhaustive scrutiny, she found no faults.

About the time Ms. Muffet had finally convinced herself that the web was indeed flawless, she felt a tremendous jolt that nearly shook her loose. The entire web reverberated. Frightened (more for her web than for herself), Ms. Muffet anxiously looked up. There, in the fifth octant from the bottom, third row down from the sixth rib across, was a large fly. He had foolishly circled into this orb of death and was now feverishly flapping his buzzing wings in a desperate attempt to get loose. These continued efforts, more than the original crash itself, now threatened to tear a hole near the vital bridgeline that connected the entire grid to the supporting posts. Were that to happen no amount of repairing would bring back the treasured symmetry. In no time Ms. Muffet had traversed the network to where the bug was trapped. The rapid approach of his deadly enemy panicked the fly. He began to beat his wings as fast as he could, but his movements only served to tangle him more in the adhesiveness of his snare. This, in turn, angered Ms. Muffet—that such a good-for-nothing, totally useless creature might accidentally destroy the acme of her persistence. By the time she reached the fly she was so furious at its intrusion that her passion increased the menace of her fangs. The fly prepared to die, only to find himself a few seconds later free-falling through the dark, enshrouded in a cocoon of sparkling floss. Arriving on the longitudes, Ms. Muffet had surgically removed the intersecting latitudes that framed the fly, and, from her perpendicular position, deftly spun replacements.

She had barely recovered from this near miss when the web received a second jolt, and a third. Two mosquitoes, drawn intently to their human prey below, had failed to survey their approach and had thus become enmeshed. In their obsession to gratify their own desires, they had not counted on the appetites of others. Stuck in their impending doom, they simply quit and waited to be devoured. Seconds later, much to their confusion, they, too, were falling free. Ms. Muffet had saved her web once more.

Enervated for the moment, she settled down upon her legs, but almost instantly the web began to vibrate from repeated shocks as flying creatures of the night in unintended, collective assault mindlessly, blindly, dumbly, clumsily, stupidly failed to avoid the fearful symmetry. But Ms. Muffet would have none of nature's design. It was her own she intended to preserve. She literally sprang into action. A large moth in the far left quadrant was quickly cut loose. A many-winged locust at the bottom was about to rip through several ribs; it was dispatched into the black. Gnats and smaller forms often became stuck adjacently on the same strand, so that sometimes an entire intertwining section had to be removed. But Ms. Muffet was tenacious at the task, continually crawling this way and that, constantly criss-crossing everywhere at once, assiduously embodying all the stick-to-itiveness that consistently characterized her attention to her work, with never a *faux pas*.

So it went throughout the night. Some broad-winged insect would be caught in the filigree, causing a temporary sag, or, through its efforts to escape, a cicada would break or stretch a bond. Each time, however, Ms. Muffet would dart to the correct position, eliminate the intruder, rearrange the filaments, coordinate the fibers, her silk-gin endlessly spinning out more rope. Sedulously, she went on, lining up the recticulars of her lacework mesh until artist and artwork became totally one.

Just before sun-up, the air stilled, and by the dawn's early light, despite the fury of the bombardment, the web remained intact. Ms. Muffet had left nothing hanging: no loose ends, except one, her elevator drag-strand dangling, gossamer, in the breeze. And just above, and slightly to the right, a lifeless spec of derelict dirt: Ms. Muffet had died of starvation.

And on the other side of the wall, energetic, often frenetic, indefatigable Mrs. Brown stopped complaining that her family never did a stitch and, observing limply from her sickbed how they finally helped with household chores, crawled slowly, painfully into the kitchen to make sure they loaded the dishwasher right.

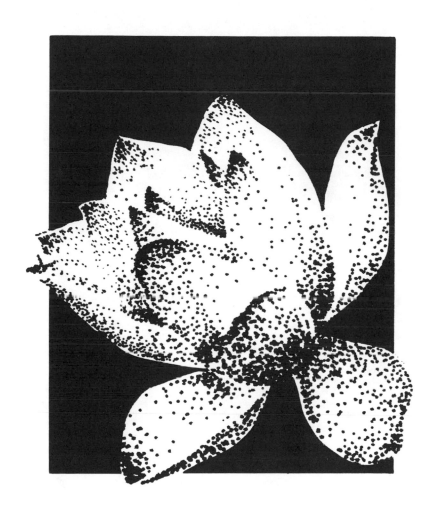

The Wallflower

Once upon a time there lived a beautiful flower who did not know she was beautiful. She possessed the loveliest petals, colorful and tender, which curled out in elegant curves so that her entire corolla had the appearance of a jeweled crown. This adornment, in turn, was nestled in a calyx of small green leaves that provided a perfectly contrasted setting. Long-stemmed, she rose above her neighbors gracefully, though not arrogantly, and the suppleness of her stalk allowed her to bend in the breeze without permanently damaging her form. Her reproductive parts also were ideally shaped to their purpose, and her fragrance was so sweet that honeybees perpetually buzzed around. Close examination would have revealed that she had no blemishes at all.

Visitors to the field always noticed her, but no one ever picked her. It was as though everyone sensed that she should be left for others to see. Not understanding, however, why she had never been chosen, and noticing that her companions, who were far less beautiful, were constantly gathered, she was filled with self-doubt. Was it her appearance? She had come to envy even the liverwort. Perhaps it was her fragrance? Was she like the voodoo lily, blessed with extraordinary beauty and cursed with a smell from purgatory? Or did she, like some poison oak or double-thorned thistle, possess some attribute that made humans shy away?

No matter the season, she never lost her blossom. This rare constancy of beauty ironically turned her against herself. For as spring became summer, and new flowers bloomed in their own nature's time, these younger flora were often quickly chosen by passers-by, thus making the flower feel perennially older and more useless, even though she had lost none of her radiance. She took to wishing she were the superficial periwinkle or some drab evergreen, and in her most anxious moments fantasized herself the innocently dangerous pitcher plant, that jack-in-the-pulpit who seduced wasps into her bosom and trapped them with her viscous nectar. Why, she might as well have been a weed: Is not a weed by definition something for which no one has found a purpose?

Then came the day for which all flowers waited: the day they were picked for the village fair. It was the opportunity to be seen by everyone. While all flowers wished for a day when they could add joy to a wedding or bring comfort at a funeral, nothing compared to being selected for the fair, where one might be chosen to grace the speaker's stand, or be honored by a part in the queen's

bouquet, or, more exquisite though more private, perhaps culled from some vase by a romantic youth to serve
as a messenger of love.

Indiscriminately, villagers rushed through the field
gathering every flower in sight, breaking them off care-
lessly in their haste. To them it did not matter if some
were damaged or others were found wanting in height;
too many were needed, the discrimination would come
later. Thus they did not really notice the flower's extraordinary beauty right then. She was simply plucked
along with many others and thrown, tangled in a heap of
marigolds, into a large basket. Luckily, none of her parts
was damaged. Two girls in a flower shop emptied the
basket and began to separate the various kinds for different arrangements. Even in the tangle, however, she stood
out, and the two immediately put her aside for themselves, carefully placing her in a special pot to which they
added nutrients and water. After she had been resusci-
tated to full strength, she luxuriated in her normal exquisite verdance. And when the owner saw her rare
beauty, he told the girls he could not let them have her.
She would bring too good a price. But, he added, "put
her in the back row," for he feared that if she were up
front, no one would notice the others. So the girls placed
her pot in the last row, up against the wall.

As soon as she saw where she had been placed,
she drooped. All her dreams were dashed. Back in the
field, when she was picked, even though she had not been
selected for herself alone, she had thought that at last she
would have a chance; but who would notice her now? As
the customers began to enter the shop, she managed to
carry herself upright, but when the first few did not select her, she began to worry again. She dimly saw the

horror of the future: left alone to shrivel, thrown into the garbage with onion skins and radishes. After all, it is one thing to go to seed in the field as part of nature's grand, eternal plan—but to wilt in a pot and be discarded with cabbage leaves and celery!

Anxious to be noticed, she began to lean forward. Perhaps, she thought, if she got a little closer to the front, people would see her petals more clearly. Maybe a different angle would help. So she stretched her stem horizontally as far as she could and tried to tilt her corona upwards to display a better view. When this made no difference, straining to get even closer to the front, she allowed some of her roots to come out of the vital soil. She knew this was potentially dangerous, but if it would help her be chosen, she would, no doubt, be replanted properly. And she tried one more thing: She mobilized all her hormones to release a particularly strong concentration of her delicious odor, hoping that her pheromones would extend her reach.

She remained in this position for several hours until, slowly, she began to realize that she could not return to her original position. She could not bend back. She was no longer supple, only limp. Her very structure seemed to have lost its organizing principles. She had gone too far. She had twisted herself totally and irreversibly out of shape. Not only that, her exertions to release her fragrance had enervated her metabolism so that she was unable to sustain the minimum energy output necessary for maintaining the vibrancy of her colors and the delicacy of her texture. She began to wilt, and blemishes began to appear along her stamen, her receptacle, her gynoecium. By evening she was crumpled, alone, except

for some fungi standing unconcerned in the darkest corner of the room. All hope was gone.

Then, suddenly, just at closing time, a slender,
scholarly man rushed in, looked around at the few remaining plants, and quickly pulled the flower from her
pot. "Just what I wanted," he said, and, without waiting
for the storekeeper to wrap her safely, paid him and carried her home. As soon as he arrived, he held her up
lovingly, and, with the tenderest care, pressed her between the pages of a book.

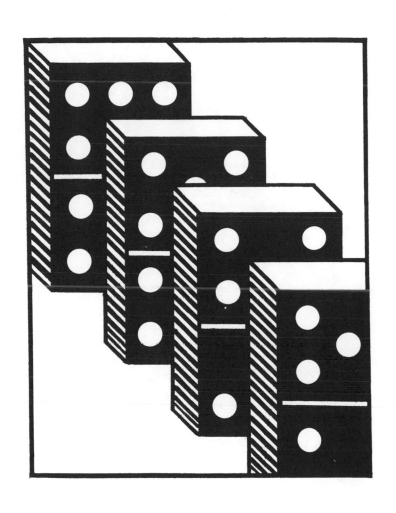

Panic

There was a row of dominoes standing equidistant in a long, narrow line that circled back onto itself. Since the distance between them was shorter by half than their length, all knew that if ever one lost its balance, all would have trouble keeping theirs.

Now and then, something happened that made them shake, and some seemed more tipsy than others, but no force that touched them ever went beyond each one's ability to rebalance, and the dreaded, unstoppable chain reaction, which each knew it was powerless to reverse, never began.

But one day it happened. It was number 10101.

Number 10101 teetered, shook, pivoted on its corner, righted itself, and then fell flat against its neighbor.

Its neighbor, 10100, was taken so unawares that it immediately fell against its neighbor, and that sequence repeated itself at least several hundred times before all the dominoes recognized the malignant state of their condition. As the process continued, some gave in without a fight. Others pretended it wasn't happening. A few became so anxious that they fell over before it was their time, so that, here and there, the tipping was being replicated in more than one place along the line.

Wherever the original tumbling order reached such a point, it momentarily appeared to stop. But the process went right on, continued by the secondary pattern. Actually, the dominoes had accelerated the process by quantum leaps.

As the wave persistently moved on, each domino mobilized all its energy to hold up or push back its falling neighbor But it was to no avail! The continuing felling force was just too much for each individual domino's own weight and size. In addition, the very nature of their existence worked against them. To hold one neighbor up would have been difficult enough, but to fight the accumulating momentum was out of the question.

The attitude of those that remained standing was pretty uniform. Each asked itself what it could do to fight this plague-like process proceeding inexorably toward them. Some tried to calculate the power in ergs of energy as against the rest mass of their own weight. Others wondered if perhaps some aerodynamic innovation could be conceived to drag this juggernaut to a halt. Still others considered the possibility that they could help their neighbors stem the tide if they could bring their own strength to greater, hitherto unimagined, peaks. And several thought of sacrificing themselves for the greater good by falling before their turn, in the misguided hope that by such action they would in effect create a "fire-line" whose gap the coming conflagration could not bridge.

But inevitability prevailed, and it was becoming increasingly hopeless to think that anything could arrest the course of these events before they reached their natural termination, when, suddenly, things stopped.

Indeed, they stopped with such resounding force and suddenness that at first the cumulative energy, redirected, created a backlash. A ricochet occurred that actually reversed the process, but without lessening its destructive effects. At some point the dominoes began to go in the other direction, straightening up again, only to fall the other way. This continued at the same rate as in the previous direction, past the starting point, running right through the original 10101, and mowing down the remainder of those previously untouched, until, once again, the last one fell against the other side of the domino that had not gone down. Again the process abruptly reversed itself, now in the original direction. But, somewhat spent, the energy being expended was just enough to push each, in succession, into an upright position without bowling it over.

This verse and converse occurred so fast, however, that before any of the dominoes had time to consider what had happened, all were standing once again erect, quivering here and there, but basically stable.

Eventually all began to focus on the point where things had turned. What had happened? Which one had stopped the pernicious process and how? At that spot all that could be seen was a domino no different in size, or shape, or weight, or color, or density, or any visible characteristic. Nor was there any prosthesis or other artifice present to prop it up or reinforce its strength. The entire line was agog; slowly each began to realize what it owed to this one member of their community.

"But how did you do it?" they all wanted to know. "What formula did you use to check it? What did you understand about its nature? How did you calculate the proper measure? What did you see that we didn't?" the others all asked.

"I'm not sure what the difference was," said the domino that had not been dominoed. "All I can say is that while each of you kept trying to hold your neighbor up, my concern was that I did not go down."

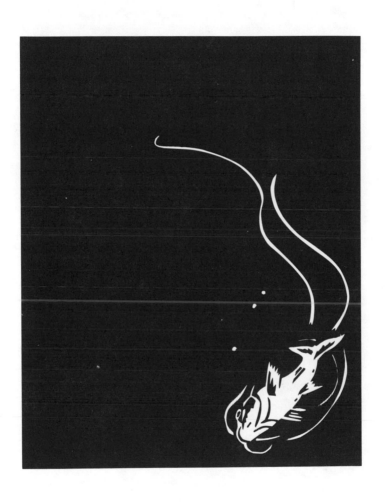

Burnout

Once upon a time there
was a scavenger fish that lost its taste for shit. She was
your normal, garden-variety scavenger and had never
previously shown any signs of being different from the
other members of her species. She lived in a normal-sized
tank with the members of several schools and, from the
very beginning of her association with this ecosystem,
had functioned in perfect harmony with her environment. She never got in the way of the others and they
reciprocated, allowing her to do her thing.

She always knew her place, the bottom, never let
things pile up, never rose to the surface unless some debris had failed to settle, and, even as more and more fish

were added to the tank, never, absolutely never, tired of taking crap from the others.

Daily she swam below, keeping the tank clean. Though, in truth, she was not out to keep it clean; the orderly environment was more the accidental result of the scavenger doing what came naturally. Nor, for that matter, did the others leave her alone because they understood how they benefited from her actions. In other words, to an outsider the scavenger might have appeared to be playing a role. This is a far different thing, however, from saying that she, or those who benefited from their association with her, ever thought in those terms. After all, one might just as well have said, "The others were there to give her something to do." Yet, on the day she stopped eating shit, the effect on the entire tank was a tidal wave. Every aspect of this living environment seemed to be affected, and almost all at once.

The first to react were the guppies. Normally a sprightly crew that glided to and fro, often in threes and fours, they seemed, on this day, unable to "stay in school." The males, in particular, normally a swaggering lot, with their multicolored tails swishing this way and that, had great difficulty staying aplumb, and rather than flaunting their customary well-attired air, appeared disheveled.

Another inhabitant of the tank that became noticeably disturbed was a small baby piranha. Its growth having been limited by the dimensions of this environment, the vicious instincts natural to its kind had never shown at all. On this day, however, ontology broke through to its progeny. The piranha went wild. With no teeth to speak of, though, it did not do much damage. Still, it began to behave in a way never seen before. Whereas previously it had moved about quite slowly,

lackadaisically taking a morsel here and there, now it swam back and forth in an aggressive frenzy hitherto unknown to the entire network. It darted, stopped, looked around menacingly at nothing in particular, and tried to bare its little teeth in a threatening manner, only to turn again and home in on some other phantom object. If this "personality" change in the piranha seemed odd, however, at least it was in keeping with its kind; not so the changes that appeared in the angelfish.

Normally a haughty type that propelled themselves about with confidence and independence, they seemed on this day to be bewildered. It was as though they had been filleted of their internal guidance system. Usually their largess provided a buoyance that enabled them to remain motionless observers for long periods of time, but now one found itself unable to remain at rest, while two others became permanently motionless, huddling most uncharacteristically in a corner. A fourth began rolling its pancake body over on its side as if to try to float, and on several occasions, when it rolled a little too far over, began flying upside down.

No living part of the system was unaffected. A seahorse lost its familiar "s" curve and, after trying to squiggle like a worm, eventually gave up in frustration and coiled itself completely into a ball; some of the more luminescent types lost their capacity for illumination, and a particularly squat and dreary-looking thing that normally drudged along by itself suddenly became euphorically friendly. Skipping a ballet about the tank, it scared the others with its sudden efforts at closeness and, on one flirtatious occasion, made a leap so carefree it nearly threw itself out the window in the top.

For her part, the scavenger fish that had lost he

taste for shit moved about, unmoved. If she sensed the changes, she showed no response at all. She kept circling in all her old patterns, but without her usual appetite; she seemed only to be going through the motions.

But the changes had not gone unnoticed to those outside the tank. One day, suddenly, as if taken by an unseen hand, the scavenger fish disappeared, plucked forth, never to return. And just as suddenly, plop, another of her same ilk took her place, whereupon the newcomer proceeded, immediately, to take up her job with diligence and relish.

Quickly, things returned to normal. The guppies regained their grace; the baby piranha again became docile; the angelfish found their gyroscopes; the seahorse uncoiled to a curve; luminescence returned to the environment once more; and the nameless squat and dreary one was once again squat and dreary. As for the previously resident scavenger, this fish out of water was cast in the refuse pile and the next morning eliminated by whoever in that system regularly took out the garbage.

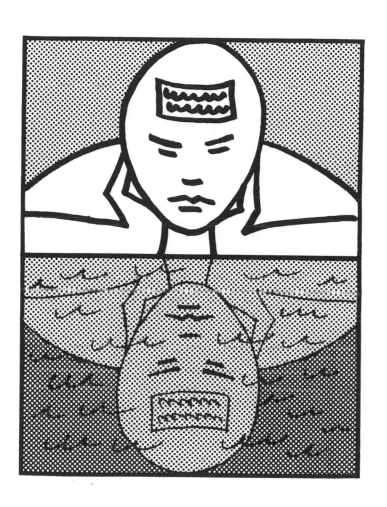

Narcissus

Somewhere around the middle of the twenty-first century, genetic engineers made a spectacular breakthrough in their capacity to recombine the basic elements of life. Using techniques originally developed at the University of Lop Nor, Sikyang Province, China, and refined in what was then universally considered to be the highest-quality proto-protoplasmic facilities on the planet (at Ishpiming, Michigan), biofabricators succeeded in generating a human lifeform from scratch. Recognizing immediately the extraordinary ramifications of this discovery, and in accordance with international protocols that delineated how to proceed in such an event (signed by every nation in the world except Paraguay and Libya), the information and technology was immediately handed over to United Nations' authorities.

After several months of careful consideration that involved the major scientists of the world, the UN decided to go ahead with a carefully controlled experiment. Under the strictest supervision, a small population of ideal human lifeforms would be created and placed on an island in an ideal climate and observed to see how such perfect creatures would respond to one another, as well as what type of society they would evolve. Picking the location was no problem. Choosing the ideal lifeforms was another matter. How many limbs should they have? How many eyes? Were the ears located most propitiously? Would the heart be better on the other side? Should coronary arteries be wider or consist of nonstick material? A cancer alarm? Ambidexterity for everyone? Perhaps the appendix, the gallbladder, and the little toe might be left out all together.

And what about the effect on culture? If another finger was added, what would be the effect on music, not just the playing of instruments, but the effect on the minds of composers when they realized the potential of the new versatility. Longer arms? What would be the effect on batting averages, not to mention the shot put? It was soon seen that each minor change in the human form could have a major effect down the road for civilization. It was decided, therefore, to create a set of committees, each with the specific responsibility for one major dimension of society. Specialists in the arts, sports, medicine, entertainment, the media, various consumer products, and various means of transportation participated, and of course the representatives of organized labor were invited to sit on each panel. Every committee was to spend a full year considering the advantages and disadvantages of changes they might suggest for this new "image of god."

Naturally, conflicts of interest arose, and vested interests politicked hard for specific emendations. Bagel makers, for example, wanted stronger teeth, and the telephone company wanted rounder mouths and flatter chins as an adaptation to a new receiver they were developing. But dentists strenuously objected to both, saying square orifices that winged out at the corners would cut in half the time it took to complete most of their procedures. Computer manufacturers wanted a "lifeport" so that there could be direct serial connection to the brain, but the neurosurgeons effectively blocked that, saying their whole profession would have to be rewired. The idea that the new creatures should come into their world with a full set of antibodies was quickly scotched by the drug companies. Insurance agents pushed hard to double longevity but were vigorously opposed by the funeral directors, and so on.

Eventually a plan was forged that, while not pleasing everyone, gained enough general acceptance so that the UN could proceed. The island was chosen and prepared with all the equipment and institutions of modern civilization. The population was to be made up of all known skin colors, with several new hues added. An optimal age-range distribution was arrived at in order to create the optimal spacing between generations. It was decided not to increase the number of genders, though limiting the number of sex organs to *one* received strong opposition from both prostitutes and pro-lifers.

Educators, therapists, and the clergy of all denominations, indeed members of all the helping professions, had been stymied about changes they might suggest. They did not see how any change in the human form could appreciably affect learning, human relationships, or emotional growth. Finally, they did come up with one small recommendation that was enthusiastically accepted by everyone.

Readouts that would show exactly what was going on in the creatures' brains, and that could be read in either direction, were to be inserted in all their foreheads. With such a simple device, no one would be able to dissemble. People would, in effect, always be "telling the truth." It would obviously have a remarkable effect on all personal relationships, from marriage and raising children to every conceivable kind of negotiation, whether in the realm of business or international relations. Such a device might hinder the playing of bridge, chess, checkers, and other parlor games, but a sliding device or switch could be installed whereby groups by mutual consent could agree not to use the windows, as they were coming to be called, for specific periods of time. In the end, despite the vehement opposition of one lobbying group representing politicians (and lobbyists), the idea seemed so essential to the fabric of human connections that all committees agreed to let the creatures themselves find a way to deal with the readouts. At worst, the inability to enjoy the fruits of mystery seemed a small price to pay for the advantages that would be gained by a completely honest society.

Finally everything was set, checked, and double checked. The lifeforms were delivered and placed in various positions, all programmed to turn on at exactly the same moment. And life began at 5:00 A.M. on a Wednesday in the middle of the month of May.

The entire first day things went superbly. Each

creature knew exactly what to do. They established co-operative patterns everywhere. Traffic was free of snarls, lines to bank tellers moved at exactly the same rate, some physicians even made house calls. There was not one sign of violence. Scientists monitoring the experiment from a remote satellite were ecstatic. Data banks whirred on. And at the end of the first day they all retired, apparently happy and fulfilled.

But on the second day something went wrong. In fact, the entire project collapsed. For as each creature woke, and went through its morning preparation, it naturally glanced in the mirror, where it chanced to notice what was flashing across its mind. And as each one began to read its own readout, it became so fascinated with what was in its head, it just remained there, frozen in attitude, and none of them ever functioned again.

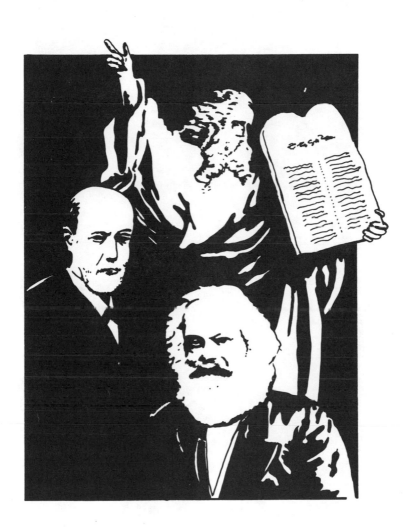

Tradition

Ⅰt is generally assumed that
once the great have passed their revolutionary achieve-
ments on to the generations of humankind, they may rest
in peace, content with the knowledge that their industry
and perseverance had turned their visions into important
contributions, relieved, at last, to allow others to evolve
their significant ideas and institutions, but it is not always so.

"Good evening, Moses," said Sigmund Freud.

"Sabbath peace," responded the early founder of
Western civilization.

"You look down. What depresses the great Moses
on an evening such as this?"

"Frankly," said Moses, "I never thought it would

wind up this way. I've come to learn how much times change, and I always knew that things would never be the same after I left. But how it's all turned out . . ."

"What gets you most?" asked Karl Marx, "the wasted resources in marble or in mink?"

"No, no," remarked Moses, "that's just a new form for an old custom. I never thought the worship of Baal would completely vanish. It's something much deeper, much more personal than that."

"So," said Freud, "even the great Moses has trouble accepting his mortality."

"No, no, it's not that. It's not the new forms of worshiping the golden calf that I find so disturbing. What bothers me is that both the new forms and the so-called improvements are being done in my name! That's what I find so insufferable."

Marx could not contain himself. "Look who's talking. How do you think I feel. In fact, I'm thinking of changing my name. With the possible exception of poor Jesus, I doubt that any one has ever had his name invoked for deeds more opposite to his beliefs."

"Wait till you've had 3,500 years of interpretation."

"Gentlemen," said Freud, "this may surprise you, but recently I have found myself obsessed with the same kind of thoughts."

"You?" the other two exclaimed.

"Especially me. They've justified so many different approaches in my name that whereas I used to take pride in jesting, 'I am not a Freudian,' I have recently found myself dwelling on such questions as, 'Was I a neo-Freudian or was I an orthodox Freudian?' "

"There you go," said Marx. "I've begun to have trouble remembering what I stood for myself."

"Well, I have no trouble now with that one," said Moses. "It's always like that the first few centuries, but after a while humanity recycles its thoughts, and you come to recognize your own ideas when they come round again."

"You talk about ideas as though they were fashions," said Marx. "Surely you don't believe it's all a matter of taste."

"Bad taste," said Moses. "I must say, I don't have as much faith in reason as you seem to have had."

"I quite agree," said Freud. "Unawareness sabotages reason."

"Don't welcome me into your camp yet," said Moses. "I may agree with you that reasonableness and love are no defense against madness, but I do not accept the conclusions you have drawn from that premise. Man's failure to act rationally all the time is not necessarily due to irrational forces within him."

"Hear, hear!" said Marx. "Moses, while I cannot accept some of your conclusions, I consider you in many ways the first social scientist. I have always felt that Dr. Freud's ideas, while useful in some applications, nowhere—unlike yours, Moses—give enough credit to the forces of society and the thrust of history."

"How can you say that?" exclaimed Freud. "Many of my major works, some of my most influential works, dealt with forces in society, and to say I was unconcerned with history—why that's just not true."

"But," said Marx, "you read history from your own already established point of view. You selected that which fit your own notions."

"Of course I did," rejoined Freud, "who doesn't? I was not a historian but an interpreter. All historians have a point of view that influences what they select and how they present it. Even the author of the book of Kings did that."

"I try to stick to facts, not myths," said Marx.

"That is precisely where we differ," Freud returned. "There are no facts, only perceptions of experience. That is why myth and symbol are so important in understanding life. They cannot be so easily cast aside in favor of so-called realism."

Moses had been observing this dialogue with delight. "Gentlemen, your differences are irreconcilable, not because of the nature of the differences, but because neither of you will permit your own theories to be disproved."

"I have no idea what you're talking about," Freud and Marx replied, together.

"Take Herr Marx's unswerving faith in dialectic. You see the authoritarian states that have mushroomed in your name as not faithful to your ideas, but they have only become caught in your own unwillingness to leave history open-ended. You set up your principles as unaffected themselves by life. Why, that's like saying evolution ended with man. After using history to make your point, you denied future history an opportunity to refashion your ideas. No wonder Marxist states tend to be closed societies. People insist upon acting out their own dialectic."

Before Marx could answer, Moses had turned to Freud. "But it is little different with you, Dr. Freud. I should be flattered by your ideas, since you devoted a whole book to me and my age, but I am afraid they have only shown more clearly the basic emptiness of reducing ideas and leadership to inner drives. The validity of an act has absolutely nothing to do with the reason why the act was committed. Ultimately, the *value* of any action depends on outside, objective criteria."

"I know that," Freud was beginning to say.

"Maybe," continued Moses, "but I'm not sure that is so with those to whom you passed down the tradition. For, when they face disagreement, their response is too often some kind of comment suggesting the other has a personal problem that keeps him from recognizing the truth. Your followers have been engaged in the kind of debate that hasn't been seen on earth since the Middle Ages. And the reason it has that medieval character is that, just as in the Middle Ages, no one has developed any external criteria for truth. Words like *sick* and *neurotic* have become the most pernicious words in the English language—under an aura of science they reck with authoritarianism. Why, the world of psychotherapy is locked in a huge theological contest. It has broken up into a myriad of sects, each with its own view of man, sin, and atonement; each with its own view of how to achieve nirvana; each with its own holy works, priesthoods and saints, sacred societies and heretics. Actually, each one sees everyone else as a heretic."

"But, Moses, you were not exactly one to listen well to critics either," interjected Marx. "Indeed, you saw those who opposed your will as being stiff-necked, rebellious, unfaithful. Maybe they simply lacked your vision; maybe they preferred another metaphor. And if you say you had the truth because the One Eternal God was behind you—talk about irrefutable positions! What's the difference between calling those who disagree with your perceptions 'neurotic' or 'unfaithful' or, for that matter, 'socialist'? In the realm of ideas, personal diagnosis always sides with the fascistic."

Moses thought a moment and then answered, almost reflectively, "I never claimed to be a great thinker—I still don't understand the Talmud—why, I wouldn't even be able to hold a conversation with such as yourselves were it not for the lessons in logic I've been taking from Spinoza. You see, as a leader I knew that my people needed salvation, and it seemed clear to me that what would have most stood in the path of that goal would be any wavering on my part—for that would have suggested that God wasn't sure. It's not necessary to believe in God in order to have religion, but religion is lost if God is seen as capricious."

"But Moses," said Freud, "don't you see that we both had the same concerns? I, too, understood how weak humans are, how insecure, how much they need order, and yet how they must first be willing to surrender some freedom to achieve civilization."

"I certainly would agree with that wholeheartedly," said Marx. "On the way over here we had been discussing Golding's *Lord of the Flies*, and it's remarkable how much Dr. Freud and I agree that civilization started with man being willing to limit himself for the greater good; but over and over some are, if anything, too quick to surrender that freedom to those who promised the most security. We have our different demonologies, but on that point we do not differ."

"*Lord of the Flies* in Hebrew is *Baal Zevuv-Baalzebub*."

"Moses," continued Freud, "you are holding our models responsible for the way that they have been interpreted. Actually, models must not be taken too seriously. That's why I argued against medical training for the psychoanalyst. I wanted the pretechnical background to be in literature, the arts, history. The purpose of a model is to permit new formulations of thought, and in turn the gleaning of new perceptions about life. I didn't claim to have invented all that stuff they call Freudian, any more than you claim to have written the whole Torah, but my followers and my detractors, like yours, found it easier to think that way. They paid more attention to my conclusions than to the way I thought," continued Freud. "And, perhaps most important and most disturbing, they forgot about my excitement with ideas, my courage to question, my thrill in becoming involved in the search. They've taken my model of the unconscious and assumed it into a fact of life."

"In religion," said Moses, "that's called idolatry."

"That," said Marx, "is precisely what has happened with the modern state. I wouldn't want to be quoted on this, but I no longer believe religion is the opiate of the masses."

"You don't?" Moses and Freud responded incredulously.

"No," said Marx, "I'm afraid the opiate of the masses now is Marxism. The state is supposed to wither; it's supposed to be a means, not an end."

"Now," said Moses, "you are getting down to basics. It is the inability of humanity to stay focused on the larger process that turns them into idolators, and that is why I kept trying to focus on the eternal."

"Do you think, then," asked Marx, "the problem is institutionalism? I mean, it's when your ideas become established, whether the establishment is religion, medicine, or a political platform that the kind of unending growth we all seem to be interested in seems to stop."

"Well, it does seem," Moses suggested, "that as soon as anything becomes popular, the popularity itself is almost proof that the idea has lost its power to help humanity evolve. No, I believe the problem is deeper than institutionalism, for ultimately human institutions merely reflect human nature."

"Why," said Marx, "you're beginning to sound more like Dr. Freud."

"We have come to rub off on one another over the years," responded Moses. "What I was getting to was that the problem lies in the leadership of our estates, the priesthoods, if you will, among our respective followers, whether they are called the clergy or doctors or politicians. They have all become too concerned with making people feel good, like my brother Aaron, rather than with increasing their threshold for pain."

"You've hit the mark," said Freud. "I am appalled at how psychotherapy has been reduced to nothing but a technique for some, and for others merely a new form of religion. Oh, I'm sorry Moses, I didn't mean that . . . that is, when I used the term *religion* I was thinking about . . ."

"That's quite all right," said Moses. "I myself am looking for a new word to replace *religion* so that I can reclaim my original ideas."

"But I quite agree with you, Moses," continued Freud. "The problem has much to do with the way the priesthoods—to use your word—function. As many people have been done in by the anxiety of their therapist as by the problem they originally came in about. It seems to me, however, that the problem has an interrelational aspect. In therapy the contract between layman and priest, that is to say, patient and therapist, is paradoxical. For the patient comes in, says, 'I want you to help me with such and such a problem, I will pay you your fee, but'— and this part is rarely stated—'I'm going to do everything I can to prevent you from succeeding.' "

"The political contract is identical," said Marx. "Once having been chosen, the leader who took the office precisely because he thought he understood the problem, and who promised to solve the problem and who was elected because of his promise, now finds the electors working—sometimes in concert—to sabotage his plans. This is obviously true in the democracies, but it's equally true in the presidium."

"Ah," said Moses, "how true; believe me, I speak from experience. Imagine having to beg people to stand up for freedom. But, actually, the clergy of today are in the same bind when they try to lead the flock that selected them out of their slavery and idolatry. What we three had in common, I guess, is that each of us tried to establish a system of salvation that would counter illusion, and those who came after us, leaders and followers, priests and laymen, converted our very systems into illusions themselves."

"Well, maybe," said Marx, "we were just ahead of our time."

"Let me tell you something, Herr Marx," said Moses, "and you, too, Dr. Freud—if any of us were to go back today and speak as we had when we were there, we'd still be ahead of our time. But it's getting late, I have to go."

"Of course," said Freud, "services must begin very soon."

"Oh, that's not where I'm going!" exclaimed Moses.
"You're not?" asked Freud and Marx.

"No," said Moses, "I'm going over to see Spinoza. We've been working on a plan to deal with all this. He's been helping me write a treatise, or perhaps it should be called a petition. We're going to publish it and call on every one of the world's religious founders to sign. We've already spoken to the Buddha, Lao-tze, Jesus, Confucius, and Zoroaster."

"Wow," said Marx, "I love manifestos. What does it say?"

"Basically, it asks anyone who has ever started a tradition to disavow completely all followers. It may not change anything, and it will drive the popes, the lamas, and the kosher butchers up the wall, but at least it will keep the lines straight, and it will enable those who want to be true leaders to get a fresh start. We hadn't thought of nonreligious leaders, but after our conversation here I can see nothing wrong with including the originators of other systems of salvation."

"Where do I sign?" asked Marx.

"Ah," said Freud, as he reached for his pen, "because I was a contemporary of Einstein, many who came in my century saw me as the Einstein of psychotherapy, but, as time will tell, I was more like the Copernicus."

Epilogue

Characters as Coauthors

えひ えひ えひ えひ えひ えひ えひ

BABY-BIRD: What's happening?

LITTLE JOHN: The publisher's throwing a party.

TIGER: Who's idea was that?

LAMB: I'll give you one guess.

BACTERIUM: Think *He* really understands us?

VIRUS: Do you?

CATERPILLAR: Well, I understand your story. It's mine I can't figure out.

DOMINO: That's the way we all feel. Everyone understands everyone else's but not their own.

ADAM: You think *He* did it this way on purpose?

MAN ON THE BRIDGE: I don't know about that, but I do know I've had enough rope burn.

DANGLING MAN: Maybe we're all accidents.

MAN ON THE BRIDGE: By the way, what did you do after you hit the water?

DANGLING MAN: At first I said to myself, "I guess you win some and you lose some." Then I swam to shore, got another rope, and went back to wait for the next passer-by.

TENNIS HUSBAND: Another dangler; you'd get on well with my wife.

EVE: Did you ever get her to hit it back to you?

TENNIS HUSBAND: *(looking around to make sure no one hears)* Nope.

MRS. K: You mean she wins every match?

NARCISSUS: I want *Him* to give me more meaning.

FAUST: You have to look inside of yourself.

NARCISSUS: Are you kidding?

OEDIPUS: "The unexamined life is not worth living."

NARCISSUS: Maybe so, but the overexamined one sure ain't worth a damn either.

FLOWER: All I want is a different ending.

MAGIC-RING WOMAN: Me, too.

CASSANDRA: A different version will be worse.

FLY: I want *Him* to put a hole in the window so I can get free.

MOTH: That would only work till you found another window.

MS. MUFFET: Listen, why don't you both come over to my place afterwards?

FLY AND MOTH: Only if you keep trying for perfection.

LAMB: I want to be a tiger.

TIGER: I want to be a pirhana.

JANE: I want to be Jean.

JEAN: I want to be Jane.

BOUND WOMAN: I never asked to be conceived.

MAROONED MAN: That's one choice you never get.
SCAVENGER FISH: What really burned me out was *His* sca-
talogical eschatology.

Will *He* be there?
He never shows *His* face.
Suppose there is no *Author*.
Then where did we come from?
Someone had to think us up.
Why?
You don't just appear.
Then where did our stories come from?
We just entered *His* mind.
Which came first?
It had to be the story.
Our destinies came *before?*
Why couldn't our presence have inspired *Him?*
Creation's a two-way street.
Well, I want to be my own *Author*.
But you are your plot.
Why do we have to follow *His* storyline anyway?
Your existence depends on your story.
I'm tired of being one-dimensional.
We didn't have time to develop.
I can't figure out if I was committed or compulsive.
I can't figure out if I was psychotic or committed.
He's only using us for *His* own purposes.
He made us in *His* image.
His omniscience is insufferable.

His omnipotence is worse.
We do have more chance for immortality, though.
You're right. That's where *He* needs us.

LITTLE JOHN'S WIFE: I see that you and your stepmother
    finally made up.
CINDERELLA: The marriage didn't last very long.
MRS. K: But it was so romantic.
STEPMOTHER: He started to beat her.
EVE: Prince Charming beat you?
CINDERELLA: His charm disappeared the day after the
    wedding.
STEPMOTHER: All men are the same.
EVE: Tell me about it.
MRS. K: At least he was responsive.
LITTLE JOHN'S WIFE: She's got something there.
TENNIS WIFE: Wanna trade?
BOUND WOMAN: It isn't our husbands that tie us up.
MRS. BIRD: It's the little ones.
BOUND WOMAN: Power is given in families, not taken.
MR. BIRD: How did you get free?
BOUND WOMAN: I woke up.
ADAM: That did it?
BOUND WOMAN: No. But then I told him my dreams.
MAGIC-RING WOMAN: Something tells me I'd better put
    the ring back on.
MAROONED MAN: Something tells me that island wasn't
    so bad.
CATERPILLAR: I'm going with you.
"DEAD" MAN: There's another way out, you know.

BACTERIUM: You people have more problems with close-
    ness than us.
VIRUS: Maybe they are us.

What I want to know is, is this fiction or nonfiction? I
mean, how are we going to be listed in the catalogue?

Fables are fiction.
That makes me a figment.
Fiction can be true.
I want to be real, not true.
Why did this have to happen to me?
You're lucky *He* didn't put you in a dictionary.
Or a self-help manual.
But there's no central thesis.
Maybe a bibliography would help.
But why did *He* pick this form?
Would you have preferred pornography?
We're all cameos, sketches, vignettes.
A legend is one thing, but who wants to be a yarn?
Its better than being a saga.
. . .or a synopsis.
I had hoped for more adventure.
I'd have preferred opera.
How about a novel? Then you get to see life's complex-
    ity.
There was no stream-of-consciousness.
It's not the form, it's *His* style.
You're deconstructionist?
Not *His* syntax, *His* slant. *He's* always leaving us to fend
    for ourselves.

Why didn't *He* use more deus ex machina?
Still, it's better than symbolism.
I want certainty.
He's a fabulist, not a scientist.
What's *He* trying to say, anyway?
That questions are more important than answers.
Then why doesn't *He* just come right out and say it?
Then *He* wouldn't be saying it.
All I know is *His* thoughts are not my thoughts.
Maybe, but your thoughts are always *His* thoughts.
Perhaps it's not our experience that counts but the staying power of the tale.
You think we'll really be remembered?
Form is fate.

MAN ON THE BRIDGE: How did it go?
MOSES: Terribly.
OEDIPUS: Did you disavow all followers?
FREUD: As one.
DOMINO: Then, what happened?
MARX: They told us we were out of date.
FREUD: Irrelevant!
FAUST: Didn't you tell them you started it all?
MOSES: They said it's the succeeding generations that create the tradition.
CASSANDRA: Then there were no followers at all?
MARX: There were plenty of followers; but we couldn't tell who belonged to whom.
CINDERELLA: What do you mean?

FREUD: Everyone was following everyone else's tradition, using everyone else's language. Moses thought he was going into a synagogue, and it turned out to be group therapy; I went to a lecture on the ego and the id, and it turned out to be an Easter sunrise mass; and when Marx saw a huge billboard advertising *"The Proletariat,"* it turned out to be a rock group.

MS. MUFFET: So the whole effort was a waste.

MARX: Not completely; we did learn something for the future.

SCAVANGER FISH: What's that?

MOSES, FREUD, AND MARX: If you want to preserve your ideas, keep them to yourself.

Why do I always feel guilty?

He's not judging us.

Then why is *He* punishing us?

We're cursed, doomed, determined.

I want forgiveness, grace.

You're sure not appreciative.

He gave us our existence, created us out of nothing.

I disagree; we simply popped into *His* head.

But *He* shaped us.

Sure, *He* gave us talent without motivation.

. . . and intelligence without discipline.

. . . and ability without ambition.

. . . and leadership without stamina.

. . . and beauty without confidence.

. . . and attractiveness without integrity.

Creation is always autobiography.

The apple doesn't fall far from the tree.

Everyone has their tragic flaw.

I don't mind being flawed, but why do I always have to be tragic?

I don't mind being tragic, but why do I always have to be flawed?

Suppose *He* doesn't know where *He's* going.

Suppose there's more than one *Author*.

That would certainly explain the inconsistencies.

Maybe *He's* not really in charge.

You mean we're not the final draft?

Let's petition *Him*.

What would we say?

We could ask for a sequel, or different endings.

It's not the endings that are intolerable; it's the ambiguity.

We'll ask for the right to choose our own form of existence.

Do you think *He'd* really pay attention?

He has to.

How can you be so sure?

Can't you see? We're still on *His* mind.

Who will go for us?

Moses has had experience with an *Author*.

He says it's more difficult now. You have to go through several assistants, and you have to fill out a form stating your purposes, and it's got to pass several

levels of approval, and sometimes the forms are
lost, and then you have to start over, or they say
you didn't fill it out right, or . . .

AUTHOR: Guess who's coming to plead for his people
again?
SATAN: What kind of deal you gonna cut this time?
AUTHOR: I'm going to give them what they want.
SATAN: More manna?
AUTHOR: More freedom.
SATAN: But you'll lose your authority.
AUTHOR: The key is not in the story.
SATAN: It's in the character, then?
AUTHOR: No, you devil, it's in the interpretation; it's all
in the interpretation.